SECRETS OF
MASSAGE

CATHY MEEUS &
BHAVESH T. JOSHI

IVY PRESS

First published in the UK in 2017 by
Ivy Press
An imprint of The Quarto Group
The Old Brewery, 6 Blundell Street
London N7 9BH, United Kingdom
T (0)20 7700 6700 F (0)20 7700 8066
www.QuartoKnows.com

British Library Cataloguing-in-Publication Data
A catalogue record for this book is available from the British Library

ISBN: 978-1-78240-465-1

This book was conceived, designed and produced by
Ivy Press
58 West Street, Brighton BN1 2RA, United Kingdom
Publisher: Susan Kelly
Creative Director: Michael Whitehead
Art Director: Wayne Blades
Editorial Director: Tom Kitch
Designers: Mark Hudson & Ginny Zeal
Photographer: Clive Streeter
Models: Hugo Baltazar, Sylwia Dziczkowska, Stephanie O'Hara,
Edd Lawrence & Madaleen Swanepoel
Hair & Mak-up Lindsey Poole
Illustrator: Louis Mackay
Assistant Editor: Jenny Campbell

Printed in China

10 9 8 7 6 5 4 3 2 1

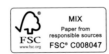

MIX
Paper from
responsible sources
FSC® C008047
FSC
www.fsc.org

Note from the publisher
Although every effort has been made to ensure that the information
presented in this book is correct, the authors and publisher cannot be
held responsible for any injuries which may arise.

Cover image: Shutterstock/Shokultd

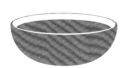
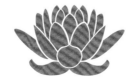

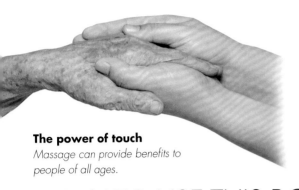

The power of touch
*Massage can provide benefits to
people of all ages.*

HOW TO USE THIS BOOK

This book comprises eight chapters. The first charts the history of the use of massage over the course of human history, describing the variety of contexts in which this therapy has been used to boost health. The book goes on to describe the benefits of massage for different body systems. Subsequent chapters provide the basic guidance you need before you start to give massage, from preparing yourself mentally and physically to setting up the massage environment. Clear instructions are given on the most common strokes used. This is followed by a chapter devoted to step-by-step instructions for a full-body massage. The final chapters special massage routines that focus on specific areas of the body, sports massage, and guidance on self-massage techniques.

Safety

While the information presented within the pages of this book is useful to anyone considering learning about massage, it is important to understand that it is not a substitute for instruction from a qualified massage teacher.

Do not give a massage to anyone with a medical condition or a pregnant woman during the first trimester before first consulting with a qualified medical practioner.

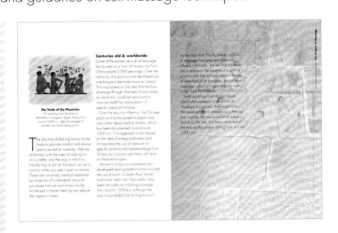

Background
The first chapter of the book looks at the history of massage.

Preparation

Clear, practical guidance is provided on how to set up the area in which you intend to perform massage.

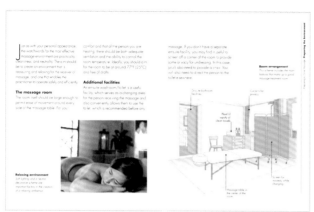

Essential techniques

Each of the major massage strokes is described in detail to enable you to incorporate these techniques into your massage routines.

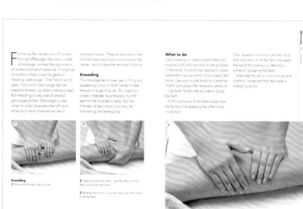

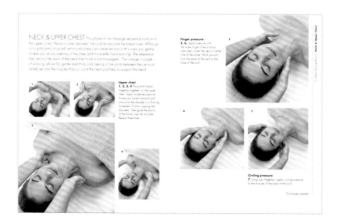

Massage routines

Comprehensive illustrated step-by-step instructions are given for a full-body massage, sports massages, and for massages of specific areas of the body.

Introduction

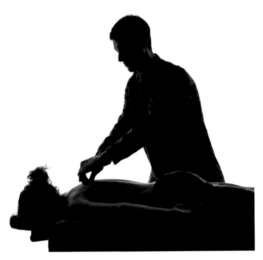

Healing touch
Massage provides health benefits for both body and mind.

Massage is an ancient therapy with a history going back as far as that of humanity itself. Yet it is very much part of the therapeutic armory available to health practitioners in the modern world. There is a growing interest in the way massage can be used to treat not only a whole range of musculoskeletal problems but also those conditions brought on by stress. It is well understood that the mind and body are inextricably connected and massage is a therapy that works on both.

An accessible therapy

The application of comforting touch is a gift we can all give to a person who is in physical or emotional pain. All of us can perform this type of informal massage. However, by extending your knowledge of the theory and practice of massage, you can make the touch you give more effective and focused on the specific needs of the person receiving the contact.

Using your skills

This book is intended as an introduction to the theory and techniques used by professional massage therapists. You can use it to enhance the informal massages you give to friends and family. But it can also serve as an introduction for those who may wish to embark on more formal training as a massage professional. Whatever your reasons, be sure to read and observe all the cautions given and remember that massage is intended to be a life-enhancing experience for both the giver and receiver of massage. Use your newfound skills with respect and care and you and the people you treat will benefit hugely.

A Two-Way Street

Properly performed massage is likely to be a positive experience for those who receive it. What may be less commonly appreciated are the benefits for the giver of massage. The process involves a similar kind of stress-relieving mindfulness to that achieved through meditation and there can be immense satisfaction in knowing that your touch is providing comfort and healing to the person you are treating.

THE TRADITION OF MASSAGE

Massage is a therapeutic practice that has origins as old as humanity. In this chapter you will discover how it has been employed as a formal healing therapy since ancient times in diverse cultures around the world, from Classical Rome to Imperial Japan, and how through the work of key pioneering practitioners it has become an established element of the natural healing therapies that are increasingly being used today alongside orthodox medicine. Massage is a living and evolving therapy, whose practitioners are constantly developing their methods to incorporate new wisdom from both conventional medical science and other forms of natural healing.

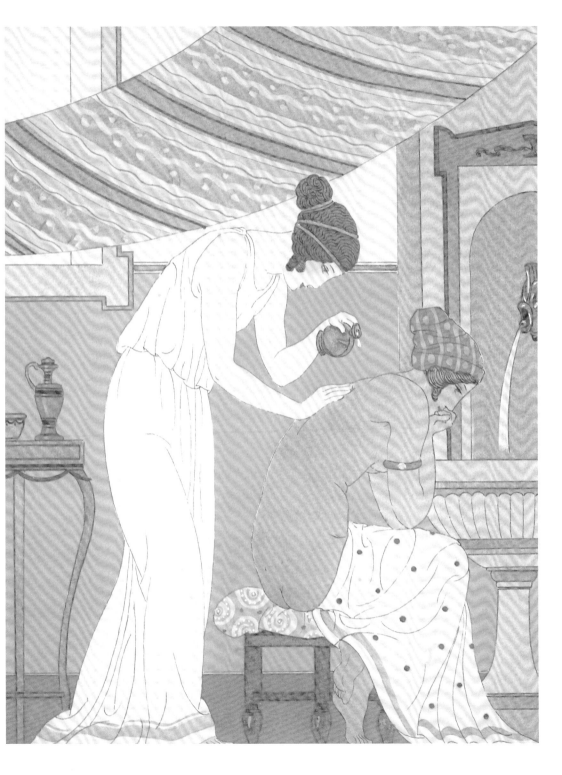

The Origins of Massage

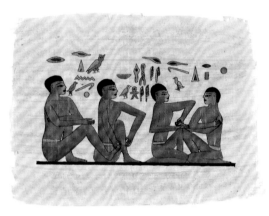

The Tomb of the Physician

This painting from the tomb of Akmanthor in Saqqara, Egypt, dating from around 2400 BCE, depicts massage of the feet and hands taking place.

The practice of placing hands on the body to provide comfort and relieve pain is as old as humanity. We are all familiar with the idea of rubbing an injury better, and the way in which a friendly hug or pat on the back can be a comfort when you are in pain or distress. These are not simply habitual responses but arise out of fundamental physical processes that we now know can be harnessed to hasten healing and reduce the impact of stress.

Centuries old & worldwide

Some of the earliest records of massage being used as a form of therapy are from China around 5,000 years ago. Over the centuries, this practice was developed as a technique to become known as "anma." This was based on the idea that the flow of energy through channels, known today as meridians, could be optimized to improve health by manipulation of specific areas of the body.

Over the ensuing millennia, the Chinese practice of anma spread to Japan and was further developed as shiatsu, which has been documented since around 1000 BCE. This approach is also based on the idea of energy pathways and incorporates the use of pressure on specific points to manipulate energy flow. Shiatsu as it is practiced today still relies on these techniques.

Ancient civilizations elsewhere also developed healing traditions that involved the use of touch. In South Asia, Indian traditional medicine—Ayurveda—has been recorded as including massage from around 1500 BCE, although the practice probably has its origins much earlier than that. The Ayurvedic tradition of massage has long used base oils infused with herbs, spices, and aromatic oils to enhance the benefits of touch—a practice that has echoes today in the use of essential oils in massage. Indian head massage, which is hugely popular today, arises from this tradition.

Tomb paintings from Ancient Egypt show what appears to be a form of massage in progress. And in particular, the development of reflexology, a therapy that involves the manipulation of specific points on the feet, has been attributed to the Ancient Egyptians, dating from around 2500 BCE.

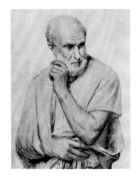

The Father of modern medicine
The leading physician of Ancient Greece, Hippocrates, was an exponent of an early form of massage.

MASSAGE IN THE WEST
The type of physical therapy that we now know as massage became a part of health practice from about 700 BCE. It was valued by the Ancient Greek physician Herodicus and his student Hippocrates in the fifth century BCE, and the Romans followed this tradition.

Massage in ancient Rome
Galen, the most celebrated of Roman physicians, referred to the importance of massage for health, and those who visited the Roman baths, including gladiators, would often benefit from massage for alleviating muscle stiffness and soreness. Julius Caesar is famously said to have enjoyed a daily massage.

Massage in the Renaissance
Along with much Classical learning that seemed to be lost after the fall of Rome, Renaissance scholars appear to have rediscovered massage during the sixteenth century. For example, the great French barber-surgeon Ambroise Paré (c.1510–90) advocated the use of massage for rehabilitation.

Greek massage
In this marble relief from the fifth century BCE, a physician—possibly Asclepius or Hippocrates— is depicted performing massage on a patient.

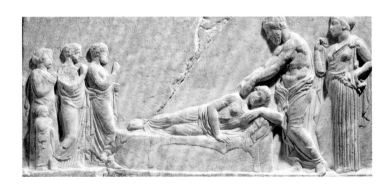

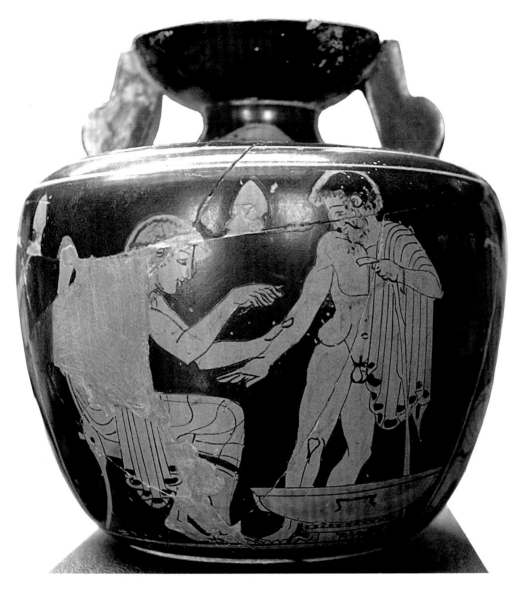

Quick fix

In this image, painted on a Greek vase from around 370 BCE, a physician is shown placing hands on a standing patient—possibly a soldier or an athlete— providing what might be instant relief for an injury.

Massage in the Modern Era

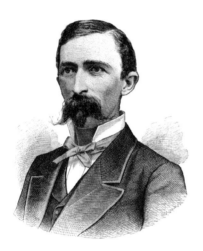

American exponent
John Harvey Kellogg, pictured here as a young man, was an influential exponent of the value of massage as a health therapy.

Many sources trace the story of massage as we know it today back to Per Henrik Ling (1776–1839), the son of a Swedish clergyman. Often mistakenly dubbed the father of Swedish massage, Ling was more concerned with the teaching of gymnastic movements, which he believed to be the key to health and well-being.

Swedish massage

However, his work in the early nineteenth century can be said to set the scene for the later work of the practitioner who truly established the principles of the practice we know today as Swedish, or classic massage, the Dutch physician Johann Georg Mezger (1838–1909; illustrated on the facing page). In his practice, he developed and defined the four basic strokes of classic massage: effleurage, petrissage, friction, tapotement, later followed by vibration.

John Harvey Kellogg

By the late 1800s, numerous physicians and other practitioners were extolling the benefits of this type of physical manipulation. A key exponent was the American physician John Harvey Kellogg (1852–1943), best known for inventing Corn Flakes. In his 1929 book *The Art of Massage*, Kellogg applied up-to-date understanding of anatomy and physiology to an explanation of the effects and benefits of massage in a variety of conditions. The book contains detailed instructions for massaging different parts of the body, along with illustrations.

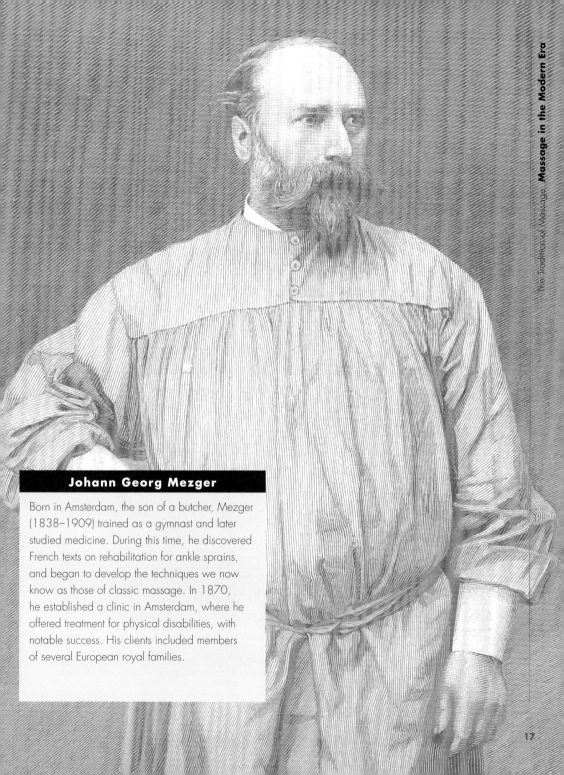

Johann Georg Mezger

Born in Amsterdam, the son of a butcher, Mezger (1838–1909) trained as a gymnast and later studied medicine. During this time, he discovered French texts on rehabilitation for ankle sprains, and began to develop the techniques we now know as those of classic massage. In 1870, he established a clinic in Amsterdam, where he offered treatment for physical disabilities, with notable success. His clients included members of several European royal families.

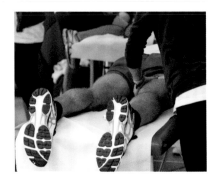

Sports massage
Today, massage helps to keep athletes and other sportsmen and women in peak physical condition.

FROM WORLD WAR II TO THE PRESENT
In the aftermath of World War II, massage was frequently used in the rehabilitation of the wounded and it soon became integrated into the training program for physiotherapists as a recognized remedial technique. At the same time, there was a huge rise in the popularity of massage in a non-medical context, as a means of promoting physical and mental well-being and addressing more minor aches and pains.

Classic massage today

Modern classic massage, while based on the principles established by early practitioners such as Johann Mezger, also draws on the wisdom of other cultures—for example, in the application of essential oils and in the use of shiatsu-based pressure techniques. The variety of massage therapies on offer is enormous—from the gentle, comforting massage that may be provided for those suffering from long-term conditions to the more intense and invigorating massages offered to athletes, both before and after competition—but all draw on the fundamental understanding of the healing benefit of touch.

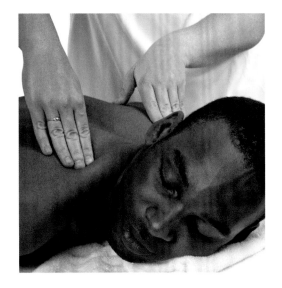

Pressure techniques
The application of pressure to tense muscles is a key technique used by practitioners of classic massage.

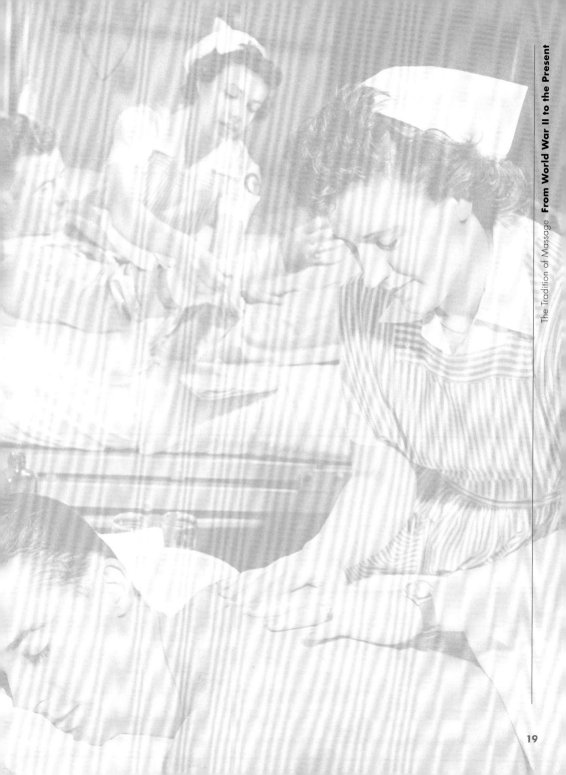

ESSENTIAL KNOWLEDGE

It is important for practitioners of any healing therapy to be familiar with the theories and factual basis for the treatment they offer. This chapter outlines the scientific and empirical basis for the benefits of massage. It describes the main body systems that are affected by massage and explains the mechanisms by which massage impacts on their functioning. Throughout the chapter there are also important warnings about the need for caution in certain circumstances. Be sure to take note of these.

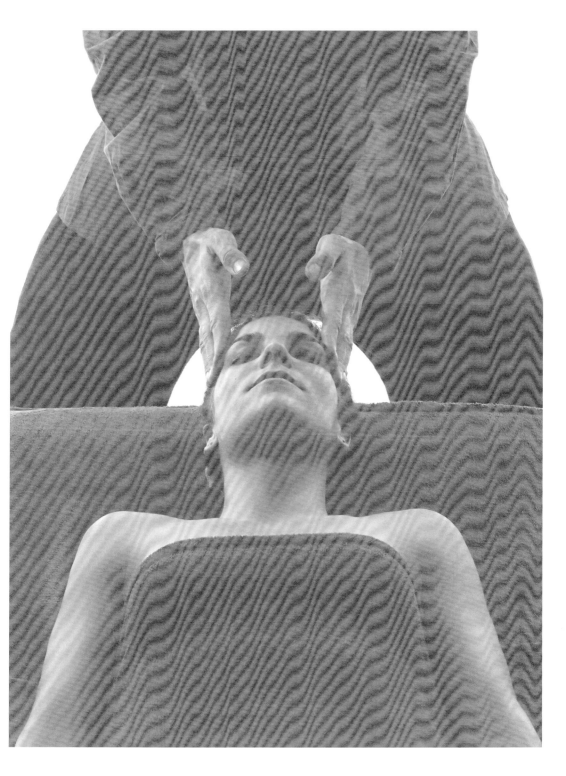

Massage & Health

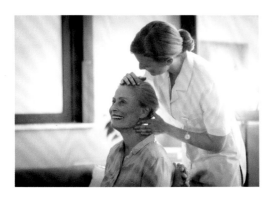

Holistic healing
*Massage addresses both physical and emotional
needs at every stage of life.*

The feeling of tension and stiffness in muscles after exercise or after a long period of sitting immobile at a desk is familiar to most of us, as is the relief provided by rubbing the affected area to relax and soften the muscle. This is the basic mechanism of massage. But its effects can be beneficial in many more complex ways, both physically and emotionally.

Evidence-based healing

The healing power of touch has been investigated and validated by key studies and experiments over the decades. In Philadelphia in the 1920s, when massage was gaining in popularity, anatomist Frederick Hammett conducted a famous experiment in which a group of rats that were handled and stroked was compared with a group that were left alone. The rats that were handled showed markedly increased growth rates and better general health than those that were not. Studies carried out between 1910 and 1935 by US researchers Chapin, Knox, and Brennemann ascribed poor development in infants in institutions to lack of tactile stimulation.

Numerous more recent investigations have testified to the beneficial effects of touch on key health indicators such as blood pressure and heart rate, along with positive mental and emotional responses. Modern scientific research has found physiological explanations for these effects, from direct effects on the muscles and connective tissues and the joints they control to more subtle benefits mediated through the skin and nervous system. And the experience of those who incorporate massage into their regular schedule testifies to its myriad benefits on numerous chronic conditions affecting a wide range of body systems, from digestive troubles to arthritis, and from depression to headaches.

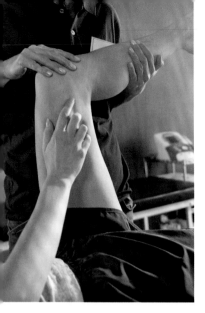

Professional treatment

Many gyms and sports facilities offer massage as part of their training programs.

HOW MASSAGE WORKS

Massage keeps muscles supple and therefore reduces susceptibility to strain and injury. By stimulating the circulation of blood to the muscle tissue, massage also has the effect of improving muscle tone, which promotes healthy, strain-free posture and ease of movement.

Muscle tension

One of the most important and well-known benefits of regular massage is its effect of dissipating muscular tension caused by many factors including excessive exercise, poor posture, or mental stress. Over-tight muscles can be painful and in the long term, if untreated, muscle tension can lead to physical imbalances and, in extreme cases, permanent impairment.

Stress-related stiffness

Muscle tension, especially in the neck, is often the result of mental stress. Self-massage or treatment by a massage therapist can provide rapid relief.

24

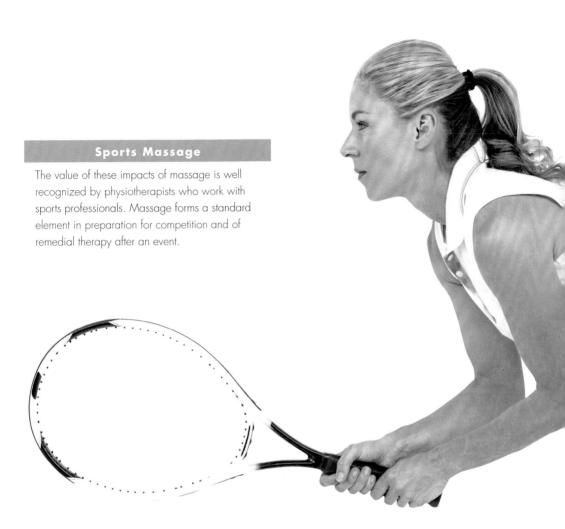

Sports Massage

The value of these impacts of massage is well recognized by physiotherapists who work with sports professionals. Massage forms a standard element in preparation for competition and of remedial therapy after an event.

Pre- & post-event massage
Athletes can use massge to relax muscles before events and aid recovery after, helping to prevent common overuse injuries such as tennis elbow, as well as providing many other benefits.

Promoting General Health

While the direct effect of massage on the muscles and joints is perhaps the most immediately noticeable benefit, another direct effect is on the skin. The application of oil and the stimulation of blood flow improve elasticity and promote cell renewal.

Fit & healthy
Regular massage can be intergrated into your general program, including exercise and a healthy diet, for optimum fitness and well-being.

Other benefits
Massage can also produce numerous health-enhancing effects on other body systems, from improving the circulation of blood to its action on the nervous system, which promotes the emotional and hormonal benefits of massage-induced relaxation. Massage from a knowledgeable masseur can also focus the positive effects on particular areas and use techniques that address specific health problems. These effects and benefits are described in more detail on the following pages.

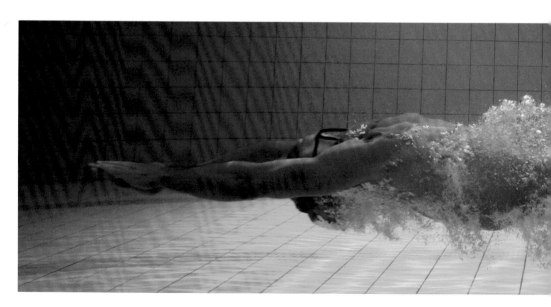

Gateway to Pain Relief

Massage can make a huge contribution to pain control in many conditions through a mechanism explained as the "gate control theory." Messages registering pressure, such as those produced by massage, reach the brain faster than pain messages, thereby effectively blocking the reception of pain signals in the brain. Such pain relief may be temporary but its effect can last long enough to permit sleep—a bonus for pain sufferers.

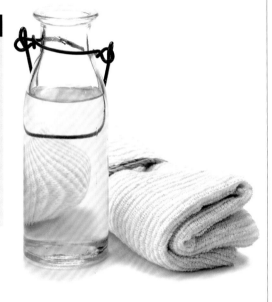

Supple skin
The application of oil during a massage can soothe and improve the condition of the skin.

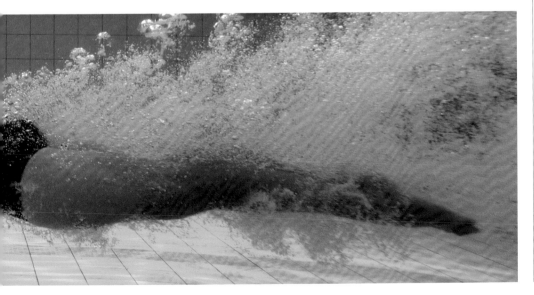

Muscles & Bones

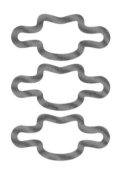

Flexible framework

Massage keeps the muscles, which move the bony framework of the body, in good condition.

Skeletal muscles are the engines of movement. Attached to bones by fibrous tissue (tendons), they move our limbs and other body parts by contracting and relaxing as needed to fulfill the actions that our brain has instructed the body to perform. Muscles generally work in pairs: when one muscle contracts, its opposing pair relaxes to some degree to allow the extent of movement intended. Even when no movement is required, our skeletal muscles are engaged to some degree to maintain our posture.

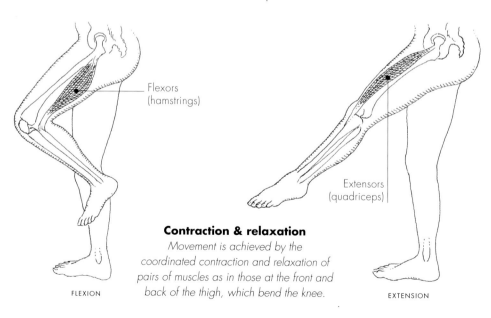

Flexors (hamstrings)

Extensors (quadriceps)

Contraction & relaxation

Movement is achieved by the coordinated contraction and relaxation of pairs of muscles as in those at the front and back of the thigh, which bend the knee.

FLEXION

EXTENSION

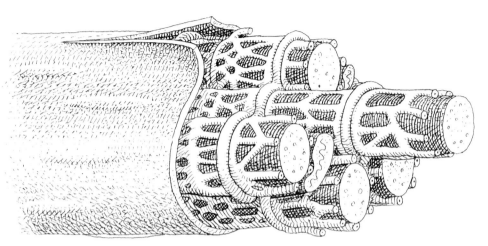

Muscle-fiber bundles
Skeletal muscles are made up of bundles of separate muscle fibers enclosed in connective tissue.

Muscle structure

The muscles themselves are made up of overlapping fibers joined together in bundles enclosed in layers of connective tissue. The muscle fibers are made up of tiny filaments that can slide against each other to contract or relax. The signal to contract or relax originates from chemical messages emitted by the nerve fiber that controls that group of muscle fibers. The energy that muscles need to function is supplied by the blood supply carried in many tiny blood vessels throughout the body. Toxins that are a by-product of energy expenditure are also removed via the bloodstream.

Involuntary muscles

There is another category of muscles in the body that are involved in the vital activities of organs and other body systems. These are called involuntary muscles. They control body processes such as breathing, blood circulation, and digestion and are outside our conscious control.

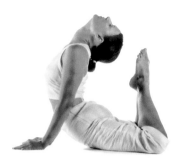

Range of movement
Massage can help to increase the range of movement possible, by softening and stretching the muscles.

MASSAGE & BONES
Although the hard structure of bones is not susceptible to the stretching and softening effects of massage, practitioners of massage need to be aware of their position and relation to the muscles that are being treated. The joints where two bones meet are also important areas that can benefit from massage. Joint flexibility may be restricted by tense muscles and relieving such tension can allow the joint spaces to expand and normal levels of joint-lubricating (synovial) fluid to be restored. This increases the ease and range of movement. And specific mobilizing movements undertaken by the masseur can further enhance mobility. There is also some evidence that massage may have a beneficial effect on the bone marrow (the blood-cell producing tissue at the core of the larger bones in the body), perhaps as a result of an increase in the blood flow that massage produces.

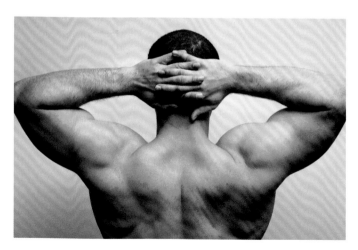

External appearance
The human body is immensely variable, with some individuals having clearly defined muscles while others have muscles that are less clearly discerned. With experience, you will learn to find the location of the muscles you need to treat.

Major muscles & bones

The diagrams on this page show the main skeletal muscles of the body and the bones to which they are attached. It is important for any massage practitioner to get to know these underlying structures to inform and guide their practice.

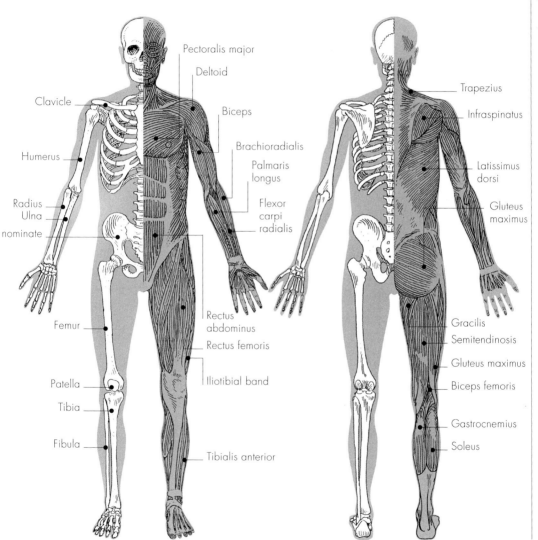

Pectoralis major
Deltoid
Clavicle
Biceps
Humerus
Brachioradialis
Palmaris longus
Radius
Ulna
nominate
Flexor carpi radialis
Femur
Rectus abdominus
Rectus femoris
Iliotibial band
Patella
Tibia
Fibula
Tibialis anterior

Trapezius
Infraspinatus
Latissimus dorsi
Gluteus maximus
Gracilis
Semitendinosis
Gluteus maximus
Biceps femoris
Gastrocnemius
Soleus

31

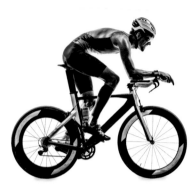

Strenuous exercise
Those who undertake demanding sports may incur muscle damage that can lead to soreness and stiffness. Massage can help to mitigate this risk.

MASSAGE & MUSCLES
One of the most well-known situations in which massage is of benefit is when muscles have become stiff and painful as a result of excessive or unaccustomed exercise, often termed delayed onset muscle soreness (DOMS). Many theories exist to explain this, including tiny tears in the muscle fibers—microtrauma—caused by overstretching, which leads the muscle to become tense to protect itself from further damage. In the long term, such microtrauma in the muscles can lead to the formation of adhesions—the formation of inflexible scar tissue—in the muscle.

Other causes of stiffness
Muscles can also become stiff without having been involved in vigorous exercise. Mental stress can lead to generalized muscle rigidity, which may become localized. The neck and shoulders are typical areas in which stress-related muscle tension often occurs. Massage is an effective treatment for all these causes of muscle rigidity.

Neck & shoulder stiffness
Massage of the neck and shoulders is an effective way of dispelling stress-related muscle tension in those areas.

Touch & Pressure

Simply the soothing touch of the masseur's hand can start the process of relaxing an over-tense muscle. Gentle stroking movements are felt by the nerve receptors in the skin, which pass relaxing messages to the brain, which in turn sends instructions to the muscles to relax.

Massage strokes involving increased pressure have a more direct effect on the muscles being treated and are usually used after preparatory gentle stroking movements. This increased pressure of massage can stretch and soften the muscle fibers and the tissues that connect them to the bone, dissipating tension. Relaxation of muscle rigidity can also relieve pressure on joints.

Nourishes & cleanses

Muscles benefit from the increase of blood flow that massage produces. This both boosts the supply of oxygen and nutrients to the muscle tissue and speeds the removal of toxins such as lactic acid, which builds up within muscles as a result of exercise. The stimulation of lymph flow from the massaged area also benefits the condition of the muscles.

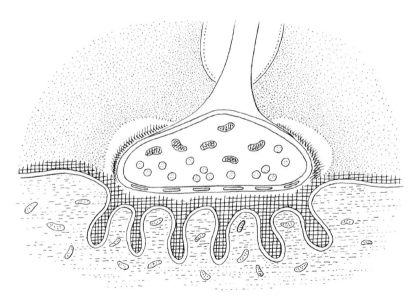

Neuromuscular junction

The nervous system and the muscular system communicate at the neuromuscular junction, where nerve impulses cause a chemical to be released that in turn causes the muscle to contract.

Joints

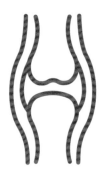

Where bones meet

Joints are where two or more bones meet, allowing for movement between those bones.

T he joints between bones are the focus of all movement of the musculoskeletal system. Not all joints are designed for noticeable amounts of movement—for example, those joining the bones of the pelvis—but here we are concerned with joints that are capable of significant movement, such as those in the arms and legs. These freely moving joints are also known as synovial joints. The ends of the bones they join are enclosed in a fibrous capsule and secured by ligaments, tough fibrous bands of tissue that stabilize the joint. The bone ends are covered in cartilage and the joint space is lubricated by fluid, called synovial fluid.

Massage & joints

While the tissues of which joints are composed are relatively inflexible and not directly affected by massage strokes, joint mobility can be considerably enhanced by massage treatment. The relaxing and stretching effect of massage on the muscles that control the joints eases pressure that can compress the joint and inhibit the full range of movement. In addition, manual mobilization can further release stiff joints. There is some evidence to suggest that massage may help to relieve painful symptoms in those affected

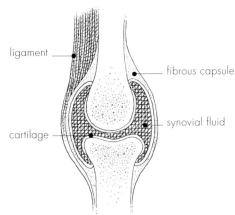

ligament — fibrous capsule

cartilage — synovial fluid

Ball & socket

A ball-and-socket joint is one in which a round-ended bone meets a bone with a cup-shaped end. The joint is enclosed in a fibrous capsule and secured by ligaments.

by arthritis, perhaps because increased blood flow to the massaged areas is likely to encourage the renewal and repair of joint tissues and replenishment of lubricating fluid.

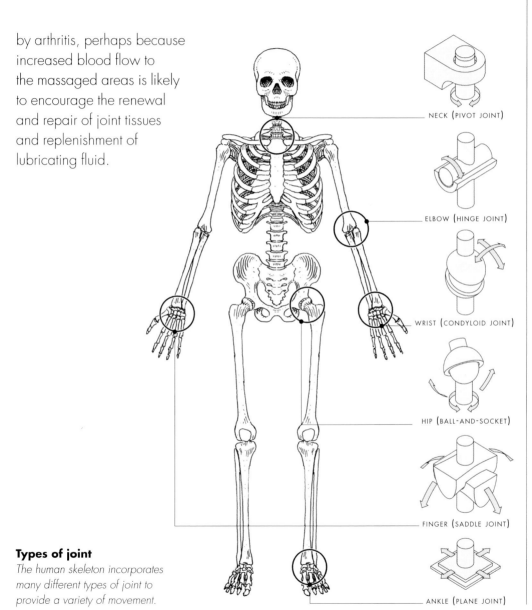

NECK (PIVOT JOINT)

ELBOW (HINGE JOINT)

WRIST (CONDYLOID JOINT)

HIP (BALL-AND-SOCKET)

FINGER (SADDLE JOINT)

ANKLE (PLANE JOINT)

Types of joint
The human skeleton incorporates many different types of joint to provide a variety of movement.

Skin

Hands on

Nerve endings in the skin immediately transmit the sensation of massage touch to the brain.

The largest organ in the body, the skin is the area that receives the most direct contact from massage. The primary role of the skin is to enclose and shield the body from the external world. It senses pain, pressure, and temperature changes, and also helps to regulate fluid balance. Not simply a protective layer covering the body, the skin's three layers incorporate a variety of tissues and structures that are of great importance for health and well-being, and which can benefit from massage treatment.

Epidermis The upper level of the skin, known as the epidermis, contains several layers of cells that provide physical and biochemical protection (in the form of enzymes and antibodies) to the underlying tissues. These cells are renewed approximately every three to four weeks. The dead cells are constantly being shed from the skin surface.

Dermis The layer beneath the epidermis is the dermis. This is the thickest layer and contains most of the active structures within the skin, embedded in cells that produce the components of connective tissue. These include blood and lymph vessels, sweat and sebaceous glands, hair follicles, and nerve endings.

Hypodermis The lowest layer of the skin, also termed the subcutaneous layer, this consists mainly of fat cells, blood vessels, and connective tissue.

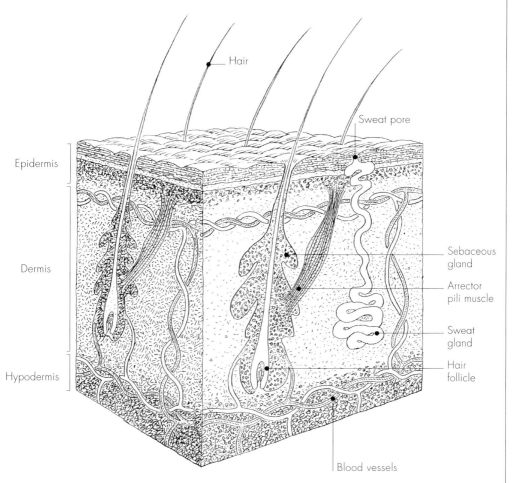

Hair

Sweat pore

Epidermis

Dermis

Hypodermis

Sebaceous gland

Arrector pili muscle

Sweat gland

Hair follicle

Blood vessels

Skin structure

*The skin not only protects the
internal tissues of the body but also
incorporates glands and other structures
that lubricate and regulate the temperature
of the skin surface.*

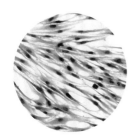

Thin skin

A thin layer made up of many different types of cells performs a wide variety of essential functions for human health.

MASSAGE & THE SKIN
The skin is one of the areas of the body that benefits most from massage. A very direct effect is provided by the application of oil during massage. This helps to soften and lubricate the skin, relieving tightness and dryness. Another important positive action is that of removal of dead skin cells from the surface. This enhancement of the natural skin renewal process also helps to clear blocked pores and therefore facilitate the flow of sebum (the natural oil produced by the sebaceous glands) and sweat (an important carrier of toxins from the body).

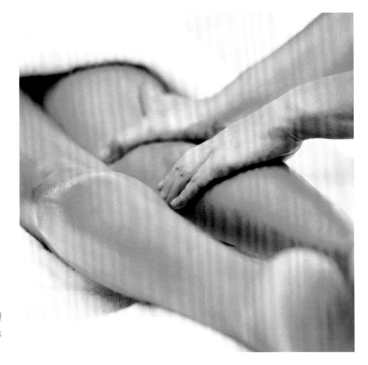

Cell renewal

Massage helps to boost the blood supply to the skin, which promotes cell renewal.

Be Safe

All massage practitioners need to be aware that massage over infected areas of skin should not be undertaken under any circumstances. Massage risks spreading the condition both to other parts of the receiver's body and to the giver of massage. Common infectious conditions affecting the skin include boils, cold sores, shingles, chicken pox, warts, and verrucas. It is important to inform yourself of the appearance of such conditions, and if you are uncertain decline to massage the area.

Relaxation stimulation
Massage can provide a soothing stimulation of the nerve endings, which initiates the relaxation process, a vital element of the overall benefit of massage.

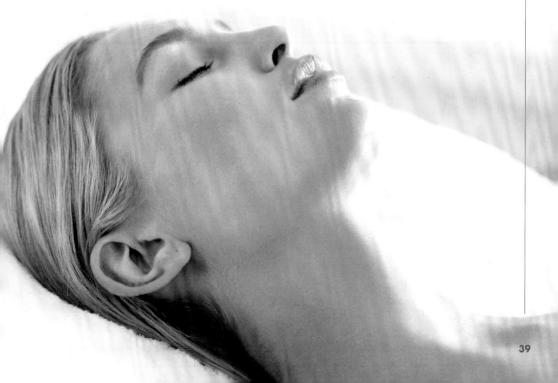

Circulation

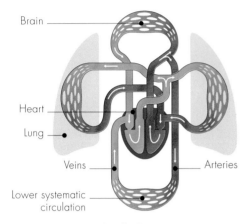

Brain
Heart
Lung
Veins
Arteries
Lower systematic circulation

Circulation route

Blood is pumped from the heart to the lungs, where it is oxygenated, and then back to the heart to be circulated to all parts of the body before returning to the heart.

The circulation of blood throughout the body is perhaps the most vital function to life. It is the means by which oxygen and essential nutrients are carried to every cell in the body. Massage has a profound effect on the workings of the circulatory system, so having a thorough grounding in the location and function of the major blood vessels will be of benefit to all massage practitioners.

The circulatory system has a muscular pumping organ, the heart, at its core and includes the major vessels, the arteries, which carry oxygenated blood, and the veins, which carry deoxygenated blood. The system also includes the tiny, porous vessels known as capillaries, which act as a bridge between arteries and veins and carry blood to individual organs and muscles, and other parts of the body.

Arteries These are tubes with thick, muscular walls that dilate and constrict to maintain the pressure that propels oxygenated blood through the system, away from the heart.

Veins These vessels are less muscular than arteries, but can nevertheless dilate to accommodate increased blood volume. Some veins in the leg have valves to maintain blood flow toward the heart against the pull of gravity.

Capillaries Arteries branch into ever-smaller vessels that eventually feed into capillaries, which in turn connect to veins to carry the blood back to the heart. These minute vessels, which occur throughout the body, have non-muscular, semipermeable walls that allow the passage of gases and nutrients into the cells.

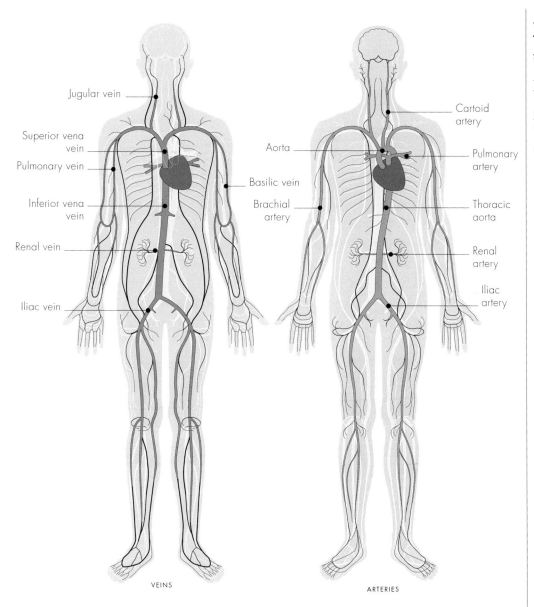

Jugular vein

Superior vena vein

Pulmonary vein

Inferior vena vein

Renal vein

Iliac vein

Basilic vein

Aorta

Brachial artery

Cartoid artery

Pulmonary artery

Thoracic aorta

Renal artery

Iliac artery

VEINS

ARTERIES

A whole-body system

Blood is carried in veins (above left), arteries (above right), and capillaries around the whole body to bring oxygen and nutrients to every part.

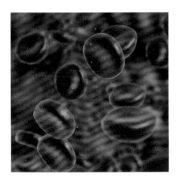

Red blood cells
Oxygen is carried around the body in hemoglobin, which is found in red blood cells.

MASSAGE & CIRCULATION

The effects of massage on the circulatory system are significant in many ways. The alternate compression and decompression of the blood vessels during a massage stimulates the flow of blood through the arteries and capillaries, optimizing the provision of oxygen and nutrients to the body's cells. This effect is especially noticeable near the skin surface, where temporary reddening of the skin in the area being massaged testifies to the increased blood flow.

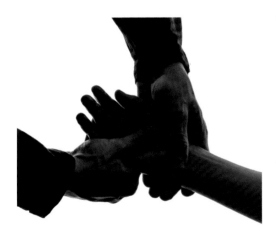

Toward the heart
Massage strokes should always be performed with the strongest pressure in the direction of the blood flow to the heart.

The general relaxation experienced by the receiver of massage, which leads to a lowering of the heart rate, is likely also to result in most cases in a reduction in blood pressure. Specific massage of the legs can also improve the flow of blood through the veins (venous return), which when impaired can cause varicose veins. It's worth noting that massage is always carried out in the direction of the venous return—that is, the flow of blood toward the heart—especially in the legs.

The flow of blood through blood vessels that are enclosed by over-tight muscles can also be improved by massage. As the muscles are stretched and softened by

Tissue Repair

Oxygenated blood flows through the capillaries. These have walls that are sufficiently thin for oxygen molecules and nutrients to pass into the surrounding tissues, providing the ability for those tissues to repair themselves and grow, as well as perform their specialist functions in the body.

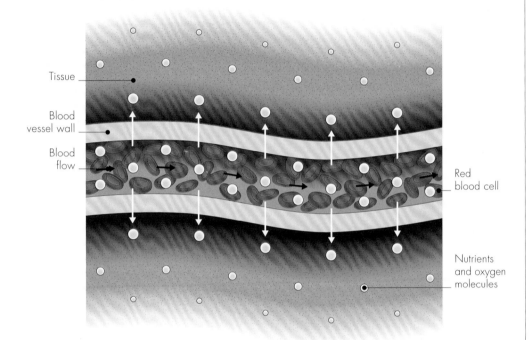

Tissue

Blood vessel wall

Blood flow

Red blood cell

Nutrients and oxygen molecules

massage treatment so the pressure on nearby blood vessels is released, and blood flow returns to normal.

Be Safe

The effect of massage on blood pressure is not a problem for most people. But if the receiver of massage is receiving treatment for high or low blood pressure, do not undertake massage unless that person has confirmed with their doctor that it is safe for them.

Lymphatic System

Draining & cleansing
The lymphatic system performs the vital function of removing excess fluid and harmful substances from the body.

The lymphatic system is a network of vessels and "hubs" (lymph nodes) that is related to, but separate from the blood circulation. Its role is to remove excess fluid (lymph) from around the tissues, along with waste particles and infecting organisms that cannot pass through capillary walls into the bloodstream. The fluid is carried via vessels and ducts to nearby lymph nodes, where specialist white blood cells and antibodies attack infecting organisms. Eventually the fluid is returned back into the bloodstream.

Massage & the lymphatic system

Massage promotes more effective drainage of lymph, which in turn aids the removal of waste products from the body.

The increased efficiency of the drainage of excess fluid can be helpful for those who suffer from fluid retention (edema). There is also some evidence that massage stimulates the production of the infection- and cancer-fighting white blood cells, called lymphocytes. These benefits for the lymphatic system are produced by generalized massage. More specialized massage techniques specifically aimed at enhancing lymphatic drainage are beyond the scope of this book.

Be Safe

Do not massage a person who has a fever or generalized infection. The stimulation of the lymphatic system risks spreading the infection. There are certain cancers that may affect the lymphatic system. Massage should not be undertaken if the receiver is suffering from this type of condition.

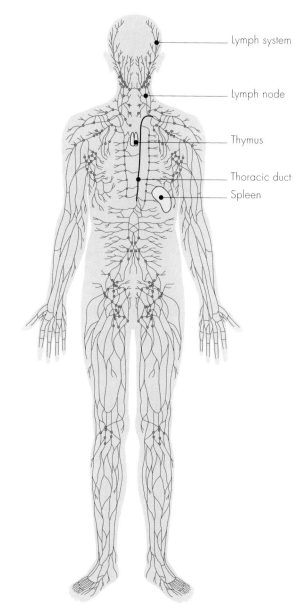

Lymph system

Lymph node

Thymus

Thoracic duct

Spleen

A protective network
*The network of lymph channels extends
throughout the body. Lymph nodes are concentrated
in the neck, armpits, and groin.*

Nervous System

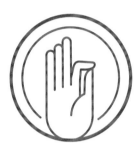

Sensing touch

The nervous system is the means by which we can sense and appreciate the benefits of massage strokes.

Stimulation of the nervous system indirectly addresses aspects of physical and emotional health, as well as directly alleviating physical problems affecting the nerves, such as compression from tense muscles.

The center of the nervous system is the brain, to which signals from the nerves throughout the body are relayed via a branching network that extends from the spinal cord. The peripheral nerves have receptors near the skin surface, which register sensations such as pressure, changes in temperature, and pain. While some functions of the nervous system are under our conscious control, such as the signals that control movement, other types of message happen unconsciously—for example, those that control breathing and digestion. The massage process has been found to have especially powerful effects on the latter system—the autonomic nervous system.

Massage & the nervous system

As soon as the masseur's hand touches the receiver's body, the nervous system's response is initiated. The receptors near the skin surface register the contact and set off a chain of responses. Soothing, gentle pressure is likely to prompt mental and muscular relaxation, as a result of its effect on the branch of the autonomic nervous system known as the parasympathetic nervous system. Additional effects may include slowing of heart rate and glandular activity, and the speeding up of digestion.

The sense of relaxation induced by massage helps to regulate hormone release, producing a sense of well-being. It inhibits the release of adrenaline (a stress hormone) and promotes the release of endorphins—the body's natural feel-good hormones. It has also been shown to increase the release of oxytocin, a hormone involved in the promotion of loving feelings.

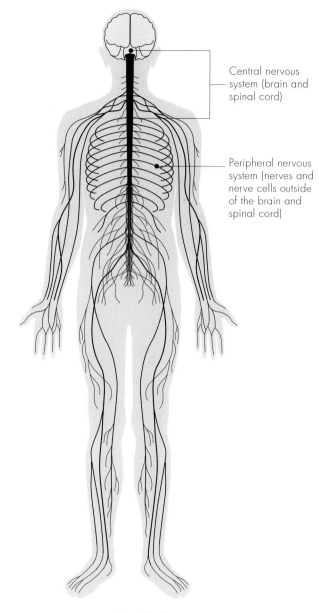

Central nervous system (brain and spinal cord)

Peripheral nervous system (nerves and nerve cells outside of the brain and spinal cord)

Network of feeling
The core of the nervous system is the brain and spinal cord. The network of the peripheral nervous system extends from the spinal cord to every area of the body.

Respiratory System

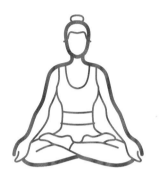

Breath of life
The capacity to breathe deeply without restriction is essential for health, physical energy, and mental alertness.

B reathing—or respiration—is essential for life. It is the means by which the body absorbs oxygen— the gas required for cell function—from the atmosphere. When we breathe in, the diaphragm (a sheet of muscle that runs horizontally through the chest) contracts and draws air into the lungs. Oxygen passes through the lung membranes into the bloodstream and is carried to cells throughout the body. At the same time, carbon dioxide, a by-product of cell function, passes out of the bloodstream and into the air that the lungs expel when the diaphragm relaxes and we breathe out. Impairment of the breathing mechanism inevitably affects the capacity for physical activity and mental alertness.

Massage & respiration

Breathing can be restricted by many physical illnesses, but also by mental stress, which tends to lead to breathing becoming more shallow. Massage-induced relaxation encourages deep breathing as a result of its effect on the parasympathetic nervous system. Massage can also ease the physical effort of breathing. Softening and stretching of the intercostal muscles (the muscles surrounding the ribs) allows greater expansion of the ribcage and therefore increased lung expansion. And in the long term, the effect of regular massage on improving posture also helps to encourage deep and therefore healthy breathing.

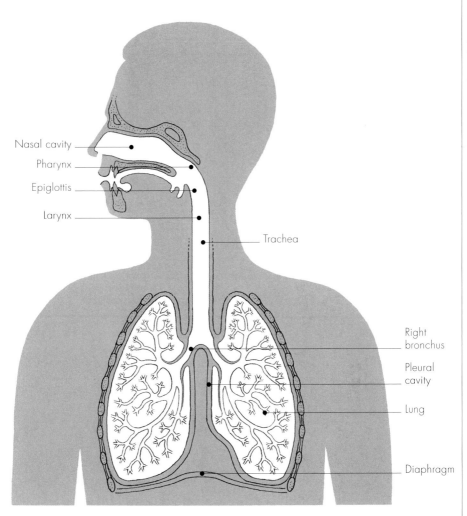

Nasal cavity

Pharynx

Epiglottis

Larynx

Trachea

Right bronchus

Pleural cavity

Lung

Diaphragm

Respiratory organs

The lungs are the key organs of respiration. Air passes from the nose and mouth down the windpipe (trachea) to the branching network of bronchi and bronchioles to the lungs.

PREPARING TO GIVE MASSAGE

There is much more to a good massage than applying massage strokes to the body of another person. A massage practitioner needs to prepare themselves and the massage environment with care to ensure that the whole experience is conducive to relaxation and healing. In this chapter you will learn how to prepare yourself physically and mentally for massage practice. There is advice on clothing and equipment, and how to manage your interactions with the person you are about to treat. Paying attention to all these aspects of your practice will make a huge difference to the effect of the treatment you provide.

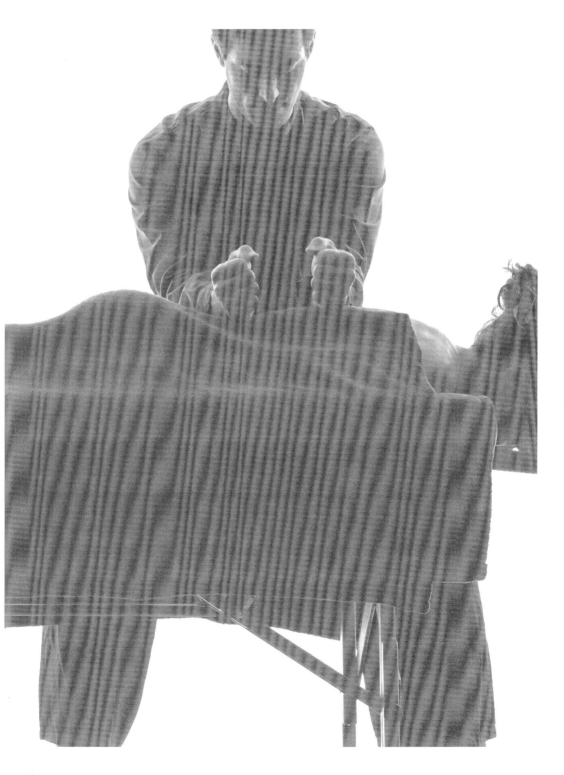

Taking Up Massage

Focus on healing
Always keep your focus on the purpose of massage—to provide benefit to the receiver.

Knowing how to use the healing power of touch to provide comfort, stress relief, and the easing of many painful conditions is an immensely valuable skill. If you make the effort to learn how to give massage safely and effectively, you will find your services much in demand by family and friends.

Amateur or professional?

Although this book and the techniques it teaches are aimed at the amateur practitioner, and not primarily at those intending to set up a professional practice, it is important for anyone offering massage to develop a serious approach to their practice that incorporates many of the guidelines you would expect a professional masseur to follow. However, it is essential to understand that if you intend to seek payment for massage treatment, you will need to follow guidelines that are beyond the scope of this book, and would be advised to consider getting further training from a professional organization.

Safety & effectiveness

The ground rules for amateur and professional masseurs are intended to ensure safety for both the giver and receiver of massage, and to provide the conditions for the optimum effectiveness of the treatment. On the following pages, you will learn how to prepare and present yourself as a giver of massage, how to set up a massage environment that is most conducive to obtaining the intended benefits of the treatment, and—importantly—how to prepare the person who is about to receive the massage so that they know what to expect and feel safe, which will enable them to enjoy the experience.

Preparatory Checklist

Before you embark on your massage practice, it may be helpful to run through the following checklist. The advice in this chapter will help you in your preparation for practice.

- Am I mentally in the right frame of mind?
- Am I physically able to perform effectively?
- Is the massage environment clean and inviting?
- Do I have all the equipment I need?

Mental Preparation

Frame of mind
Inner calm and focus is essential for effective massage.

Transmitting confidence
Whatever kind of massage you are undertaking, it is vital to transmit an air of confidence.

Massage is much more than a physical process. When you lay your hands on the body of another person, the contact is capable of transmitting your emotions and your state of mind to the person who is receiving your touch. This can work to the benefit of the treatment, but can also have a negative effect.

A relaxed and confident practitioner conveys reassurance and promotes relaxation through their hands. But massage from someone who is tense or nervous, or possibly distracted, is likely to make the person receiving the massage pick up on these feelings, and as a result feel less able to release any stress. For this reason, you need to ensure that you develop techniques for focusing your mind in a positive way to achieve the intended benefits of the treatment.

Focus & detachment

One of the keys to providing beneficial massage is developing an approach that is both engaged and detached. Your focus must be on the massage process, ignoring outside distractions, and you need to remain detached from your feelings about the individual to whom you are giving the massage, while being alert to their physical responses to your touch. Teachers of massage often describe the correct mental attributes as "intention" and "focus." The intention of the massage should be the therapeutic benefit that you are intending to achieve. The focus is on the process of achieving that benefit.

Inner focus
Centering is a vital technique for achieving an inner focus that enables you to transmit healing energy.

CENTER YOURSELF
Many masseurs find that learning and practicing meditation techniques helps them to make the transition from a state of mind in which they are dealing with everyday concerns to the more focused state that is needed to provide effective massage. There are many different centering routines that can help you adopt the necessary focus, but this simple routine is a quick and easy one to try before starting to give massage.

Inner serenity
Before you undertake massage, use a technique of your choice to exclude extraneous thoughts and concerns so you can focus on your massage practice.

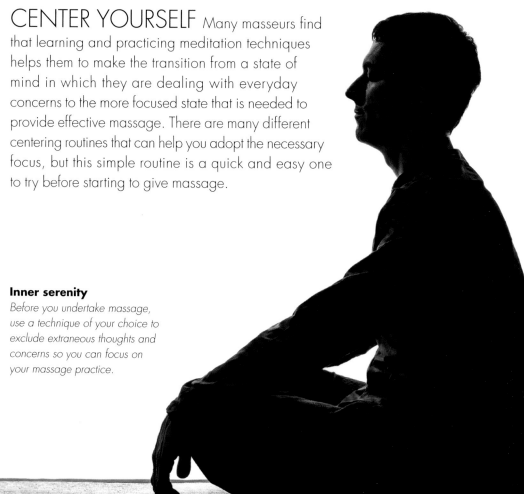

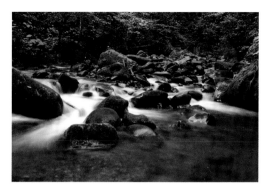

Visualization

Some people find that imagining the flow of water in a stream helps them to visualize stresses flowing out of their consciousness.

Centering Routine

- Kneel or sit in a comfortable position with your eyes closed.

- Sense your contact with the floor and the solidity of the support it provides.

- Move your focus from your buttocks and pelvic area up through your spine and trunk, allowing your awareness to take in your arms, hands, and shoulders. Let go of any tightness or tension you notice.

- Now focus on the neck, jaw, and face, releasing any tension there.

- Turn your attention to your breathing. Notice how the breath flows in and out, without forcing the process. Imagine stress and tension leaving your body as you exhale. After a few minutes of this deep and gentle breathing, open your eyes.

Grounding

You will use the ability to achieve mental focus when you perform grounding touch—a technique that is explained later in the book.

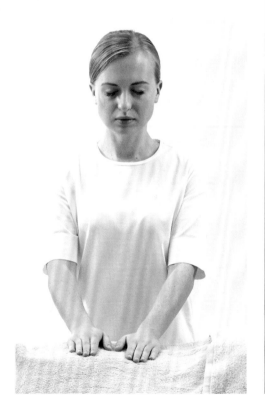

Physical Fitness & Health

Giving massage demands both strength and stamina, so as a practitioner of massage, you need to ensure that you are sufficiently fit to avoid strain or excessive fatigue while giving a treatment. You will benefit from taking steps to maintain your general health and physical fitness, such as adhering to a well-balanced diet containing a wide variety of vitamins and other nutrients, without excessive amounts of sugar or fat.

There are all kinds of good reasons for keeping your weight within healthy limits, but in the context of giving massage, avoiding excess weight gain will help you remain agile, enabling you to maneuver around the massage table and the receiver of massage as necessary.

Strength & stamina

To optimize your ability to sustain a vigorous and extended massage, it is vital to reach and maintain a reasonable level of overall fitness. You don't need to be an Olympic athlete, but it is advisable to embark on a sensible routine of taking regular aerobic exercise of whatever kind

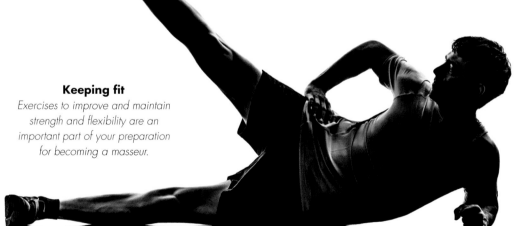

Keeping fit

Exercises to improve and maintain strength and flexibility are an important part of your preparation for becoming a masseur.

you enjoy—for example, running, cycling, swimming, or tennis. In addition, consider taking up an activity that increases your flexibility. Yoga is ideal as it builds strength and flexibility, but is also calming and contributes to mental focus. Tai chi, which emphasizes breathing and controlled movement, is another form of exercise that can be useful for practitioners of massage.

Get a Massage

As a massage practitioner, you will benefit hugely from receiving massage yourself. Not only does it address any strain or tension that you may incur during your practice, but it also acts as a reminder of what the receiver of massage experiences—a valuable insight.

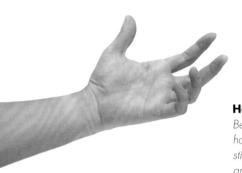

Hands & fingers

Before each massage session, make sure your hands and fingers are free of tension and stiffness, by gently moving the joints of the wrists and fingers through their full range.

PHYSICAL PREPARATION
There are some exercises that it is useful to practice in preparation for massage. In particular, it is valuable to become familiar with the ideal stances to adopt when performing massage. Using the recommended stance not only optimizes your mobility and the force and direction of the strokes, but also helps to protect you from strain.

Healthy standing posture

As a starting point, examine how you stand. A healthy standing posture balances the weight of the head vertically over the spine. This minimizes strain on the back. Be sure to keep your pelvis level to distribute your weight evenly over your legs.

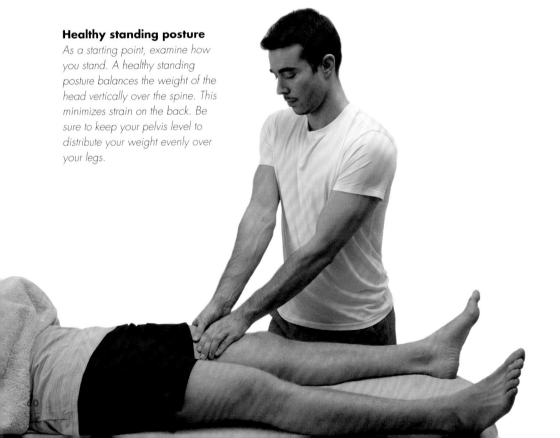

Square stance

Stand next to your massage table with your feet just over hip width apart. Place your feet with your toes in line with the edge of the table, pointing outward at an angle of about 45 degrees. Keep your knees soft (slightly bent) and your back straight. Move your hips forward and tuck in your bottom slightly. Rest your arms on the table with your elbows at right angles. Practice looking down without bending your neck. This stance is used for short strokes and working across the body.

Striding stance

Stand next to your massage table at an angle of approximately 45 degrees with the outside leg forward, with the knee bent, and the inside leg back, with the knee almost straight. Keeping the knees soft and the back straight, practice moving back by straightening the outside knee and moving your weight onto the inner leg. Then move forward again by bending the outer knee and shifting your weight forward onto that leg. This stance is used for long strokes.

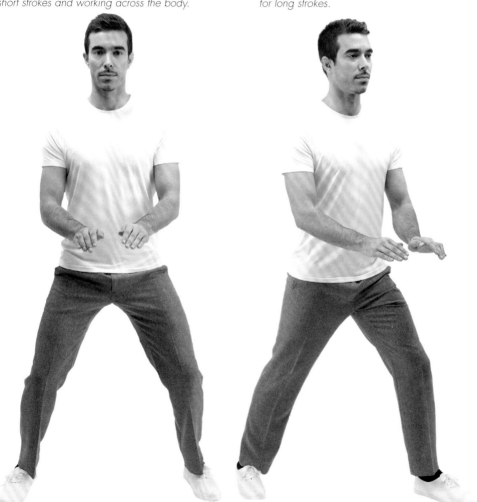

Cleanliness & Clothing

Massage involves close personal contact between the giver and receiver of massage, so it is obvious that the person giving the massage needs to pay rigorous attention to personal hygiene from the point of view of health and the comfort of the person receiving the massage. There should be no suspicion of body odor, so a daily shower is essential. And avoid using strongly scented toiletries—your presence should be as neutral as possible.

Clothing

The priority is to wear clean clothing that allows complete freedom of movement. For a nonprofessional, a loose-fitting T-shirt and jogging pants are ideal. And cotton is an ideal choice of fabric as it is cool and breathable. From an aesthetic point of view, pale colors are preferable because they would show any dirt, so it is obvious to the person you are treating that you are wearing clean clothes. Choose lightweight, flat shoes with nonslip soles.

Clean & comfortable
Be sure to choose clothing that does not restrict your movement.

Hair

As well as appearing clean and well kempt, your hair—whether short or long—should be arranged so as not to get in the way of your face while you are performing massage. It would be unacceptably distracting to change hand positions while you push hair out of your eyes. So be sure to tie back your hair securely and use a hairband, if necessary, to keep a floppy fringe off your face.

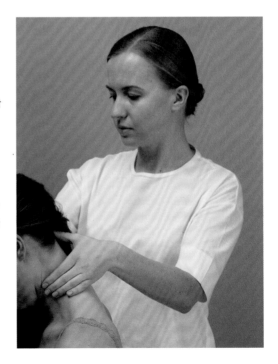

Hands & nails

Particular attention needs to be given to the condition and appearance of your hands. You must wash your hands thoroughly before starting each treatment, using an antibacterial handwashing product. Frequent washing can lead to dryness of the skin so use hand cream to keep your hands smooth and free of cracks after the massage session is over. Don't use hand cream before giving massage as you do not want to transfer the cream to the receiver of your treatment.

Keep your nails short, smooth, and well-manicured. Long nails risk scratching during massage. Do not use colored nail lacquer, which looks unprofessional (a concern even if you are offering treatment on an amateur basis) and may conceal dirt underneath.

Preparing the Environment

Just as with your personal appearance, the watchwords for the most effective massage environment are practicality, cleanliness, and neutrality. The aim should be to create an environment that is reassuring and relaxing for the receiver of massage, and one that enables the practitioner to operate safely and efficiently.

The massage room

The room itself should be large enough to permit ease of movement around every side of the massage table. For your comfort and that of the person you are treating, there should be both adequate ventilation and the ability to control the room temperature. Ideally, you should aim for the room to be at around 77°F (25°C) and free of drafts.

Additional facilities

An en-suite washroom/toilet is a useful facility, which serves as a changing area for the person receiving the massage and also conveniently allows them to use the toilet, which is recommended before any

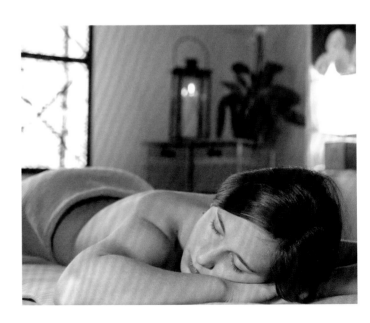

Relaxing environment
Soft lighting and a neutral decorative scheme are important factors in the creation of a relaxing ambience.

massage. If you don't have a separate en-suite facility, you may find it useful to screen off a corner of the room to provide some privacy for undressing. In this case, you'll also need to provide a chair. You will also need to direct the person to the toilet elsewhere.

Room arrangement

This scheme includes the main features that make up a good massage treatment room.

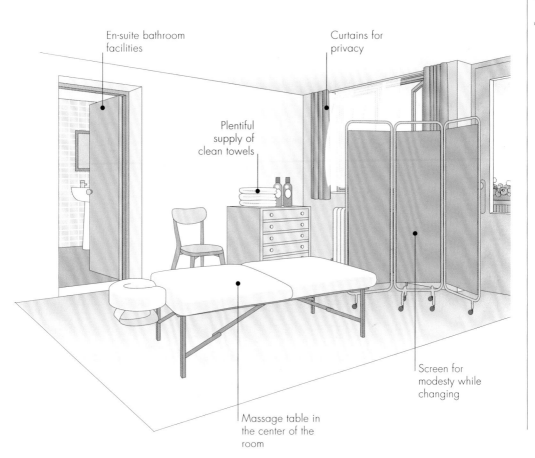

En-suite bathroom facilities

Curtains for privacy

Plentiful supply of clean towels

Screen for modesty while changing

Massage table in the center of the room

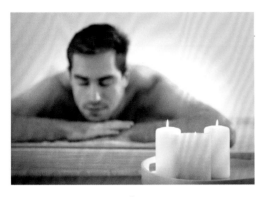

Room fragrance
Scented candles are a good way of fragrancing the massage environment.

Lighting

Natural light is always a bonus, but any room in which you undertake massage should have its windows shielded by blinds or drapes. These do not have to exclude all light, but must ensure the privacy of the massage. At the start and end of a session, for practical reasons you need to have adequate lighting to set up and clear away your equipment, but while treatment is underway, subdued lighting is generally preferred. You need enough light to see, for example, any skin problems. It is also useful to be able to see the face of the person you are massaging, to note changes in expression that might indicate discomfort. But many of the signals you receive are through touch and bright light is not needed. The receiver of massage is better able to relax if the light levels are low, and this is an overriding consideration.

It is worthwhile investing in dimmable lights, with perhaps a brighter side light over the shelf or table where you keep your equipment and oils.

Scent

The scents around us are a powerful determinant of mood, and many massage therapists use the subtle fragrance of essential oils to help create a relaxing and harmonious atmosphere. There are many ways of scenting a room, from diffuser sticks immersed in scented oils to essential oil burners and candles. But whichever method you choose, be careful not to overdo it. And be conservative in your choice of scent; our reactions to different scents can be very personal and anything too powerful may have the opposite effect from what you intend. Go for light fragrances such as lavender, which is known for its relaxing properties.

Music

Gentle sounds can create an ambience that is conducive to relaxation, but as with fragrance, it needs to be subtle and in the background, with the volume low. You can obtain recordings specially designed for use during therapies such as massage. These often contain gently evolving harmonies, but usually no discernible words. Always ask the person being treated if they find the music pleasant and be prepared to turn it off if they object.

Massage Table

A purpose-made massage table is desirable for any serious practitioner of massage, whether professional or amateur. An improvised set-up can be used in some situations, but a proper massage table is more comfortable for both the receiver and giver of massage. You can buy tables that fold for ease of storage when not in use.

Covering the massage table

A clean cover should be placed over the surface of the table. Many professionals use a disposable paper couch roll that is easily changed between each client. You can also buy fabric couch covers to fit most tables. You will need at least two of these so that they can be changed for each user. Alternatively, you may find that using a towel or sheet works well for you. Any type of fabric cover should be laundered between sessions for each person you treat.

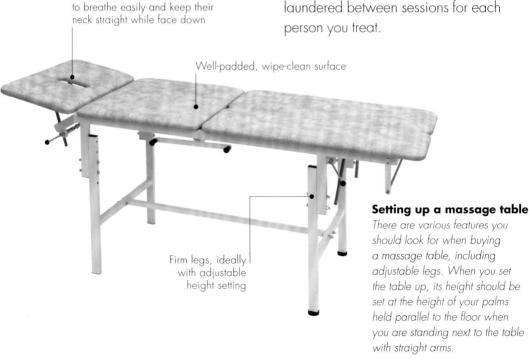

Face hole, to allow the receiver to breathe easily and keep their neck straight while face down

Well-padded, wipe-clean surface

Firm legs, ideally with adjustable height setting

Setting up a massage table

There are various features you should look for when buying a massage table, including adjustable legs. When you set the table up, its height should be set at the height of your palms held parallel to the floor when you are standing next to the table with straight arms.

Towels

A plentiful supply of clean towels is
essential for any serious practitioner of
massage. These must be changed for
each user. For each session, you will need
at least one giant towel—large enough
to cover the body of the person without
loss of modesty. It is helpful to have at
least three extra towels to hand to use to
provide extra covering or support as you
work on different areas of the body. And
of course, always keep a clean hand
towel in your washing facility. As with
your clothing, choose a pale color for
your towels to make it obvious that they
are clean.

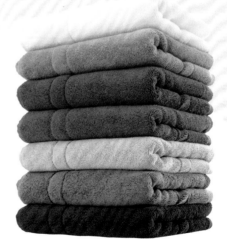

A range of towels

*A good supply of large towels is a
simple but essential element of your
massage equipment.*

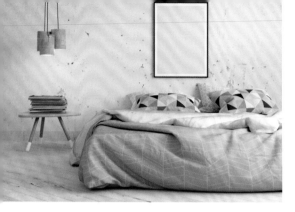

Soft surface
A bed is likely to be too soft for effective massage. It is preferable to set up a massage surface on the floor.

MASSAGE WITHOUT A TABLE
If you don't have a massage table, or if you want to give an impromptu massage in somebody else's house, it's useful to know how to set up an improvised massage area.

Setting Up a Massage Area

- Place a futon, length of foam, or thin guest mattress on the floor. Several layers of folded blankets may also be adequate. Cover with a large towel, sheet, or blanket.

- For face-up massage, place a firm pillow at each end—one to support the head and one to provide support under the knees.

- For face-down massage, make a towel roll about 12 inches (30 cm) in length and place in a semicircle at the head of the mattress to support the forehead while keeping the nose and mouth clear of the surface underneath.

- Place additional folded towels under the shoulders and anywhere else that may need additional support or padding.

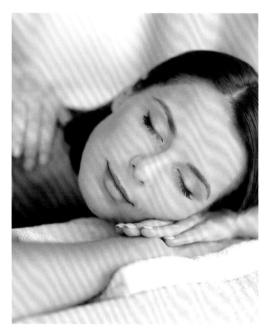

Improvised comfort
Wherever you set up your massage surface, the comfort of the person you are treating is a priority.

Seated massage

Sometimes it is best to use a chair for massage—for example, of the neck and shoulders in an office. And some people with reduced mobility may find it difficult to climb onto a massage table. For this reason, it is useful to have a firm chair available. One with a plain, straight back on which the receiver can sit astride and support themselves can be useful in these situations. A stool is best suited to head and face massage.

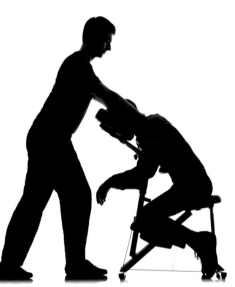

Massage chair

Some professional massage practitioners invest in a special massage chair. But this is outside the scope of most of those starting a massage career.

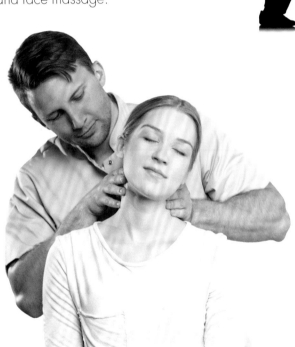

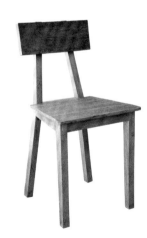

Impromptu massage

In some situations, for example when neck stiffness sets in, an impromptu seated massage is the answer.

Upright chair

A simple upright chair can be used for neck and shoulder massage as long as it is firm and steady.

Before You Start

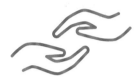

Creating trust

A friendly handshake is a perfect way of establishing an atmosphere of trust between the giver and receiver of massage.

How you start a massage session, whether as an amateur or professional, can have a huge impact on the tone and effectiveness of the entire treatment. It is important to put the person at their ease as soon as possible and establish an atmosphere of trust and confidence.

Before arrival

To get yourself in the right frame of mind, be sure you are prepared well before the person arrives for their massage. Arrange the room with a clean cover on the table and a plentiful supply of clean towels. Get changed into your massage clothing and try to find time for a few minutes of your usual centering routine. Turn off any source of distraction, such as phones or sound notifications of text messages or emails.

Setting the scene

When the person arrives for their massage, you need to start by putting them at their ease—they may be apprehensive, especially if this is their first massage. A firm handshake and a relaxed smile are important for creating the right atmosphere. Your demeanor should be quietly confident and reassuring during all your interactions with the person you are treating.

Before the person gets undressed, have a clear conversation about what kind of massage they want and whether they have any existing medical conditions or undiagnosed pain. See the checklist (opposite) and follow the advice given if the person has any of the conditions listed. Note: because this book is aimed at those who have little training in massage, the advice here is conservative. Qualified masseurs may have the necessary experience to undertake massage in some of the conditions where "do not massage" advice is given.

Caution	
CONDITION	ACTION
Pregnancy	Do not massage
Fever	Do not massage
Cancer	Do not massage
Under the influence of alcohol or drugs	Do not massage
Skin condition (infectious or uncertain)	Do not massage
Skin condition (noninfectious)	Avoid affected area
Swellings, cuts, bruises	Avoid affected area
Varicose veins	Avoid affected area
Menstruation	Avoid massage of belly
Recent surgery	Do not massage

For any condition requiring continuing medication, ask the person to seek the approval of their doctor before undertaking massage.

Explaining the Process

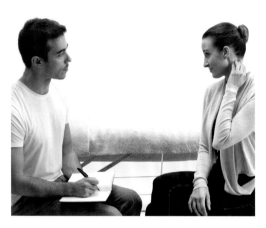

Initial conversation
Be sure to listen carefully and make a note of any special concerns that the person may have.

Once you have determined that it is safe to proceed with the massage, you can give a further explanation of what the treatment will entail. Massage can seem like a very intimate process.

Clear & businesslike

Be aware that massage has the potential for creating embarrassment. The receiver is often only minimally clothed, and is then touched on their bare skin by the giver of massage. For many people, this is much closer contact than they would normally permit outside a close relationship. To ensure that the person who is about to receive the massage is totally at ease with what is about to happen, a clear and businesslike explanation is essential.

Describing what will happen

If this is the first time you have given the person massage, take the trouble to go through what to expect in a fair amount of detail, from the practicalities of where to get undressed, and what clothes to leave on, to how they will lie on the massage table and what parts of the body will be touched first. Be sure to inquire if they are happy for you to use oils and if they are aware of any allergies to specific oils.

Describe to the massage recipient the normal sensations that massage may produce, such as warmth in the area being worked and increased activity of the digestive tract. Explain that relaxation is an important aim of massage, so they should exclude the possibility of outside distractions interfering with this process. To this end, ask the person to switch off their cell phone for the duration of the massage.

Remember to listen

This introductory chat is not simply an opportunity for you to explain about the massage process, it is also an important opportunity for the receiver of massage to ask questions, air any anxieties, and seek specific reassurances. Be sure to make space in the conversation for the person to express their uncertainties, views, and feelings. Take their anxieties seriously and set their mind at rest where appropriate.

Observing Modesty & Comfort

Those who are at ease with nudity and bodily contact can easily forget that, for others, exposing their body and having another person touch their bare skin can seem a gross invasion of their privacy. The measures you take to preserve their modesty are key to the success of the therapy.

Getting undressed

It is essential that the person does not feel watched while undressing. If you don't have an en-suite changing room and the person needs to change in the massage room, go outside while they undress. Suggest that they use the toilet before you start. Make sure a very large towel

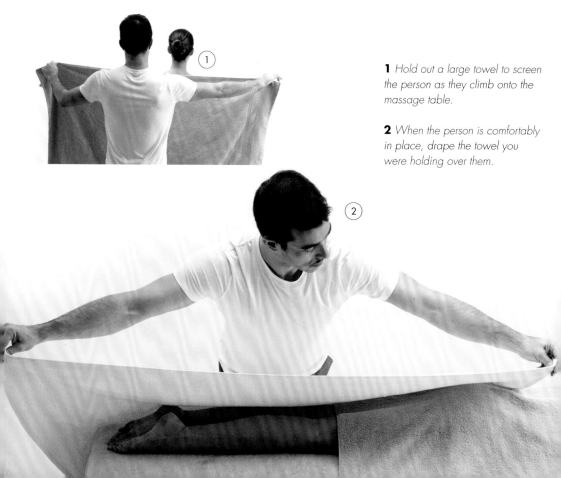

1 *Hold out a large towel to screen the person as they climb onto the massage table.*

2 *When the person is comfortably in place, drape the towel you were holding over them.*

is placed in the changing area for them to wrap around themselves, and ask them to sit on the couch when they are ready.

For a full-body massage, the person will need to remove all clothing other than their underpants. If only a part of the body is to be massaged, the person may only need to remove clothing from that part.

Getting onto the massage table

Make sure that the person can easily get onto the table. A stool can be useful if the table is too high and be prepared to offer a supportive arm. Help the person drape the towel to cover their body for both modesty and warmth before you start the massage.

In need of help
A person with mobility problems may need help getting on and off the massage table.

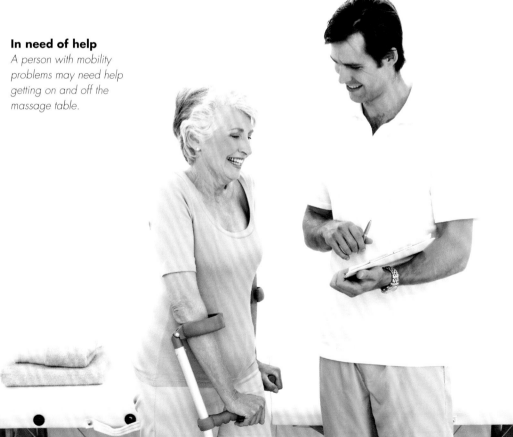

When to Stop

Massage can sometimes produce feelings of discomfort or even pain, especially when treating stiff or knotted muscles. Always make it clear to the person you are treating that they should tell you in words or by signaling if they experience pain or discomfort, or wish you to stop for any reason.

However, it is also the job of the person performing the massage to be aware of the response of the person to the strokes and the degree of pressure you are using. As you gain experience, you will find it increasingly easy to sense the changes in tension that may indicate discomfort on the part of the receiver, even if the person doesn't mention it. In this case, you can adapt your approach to relieve the problem.

Easing the pressure

Remember that there is no benefit in persisting with the massage through pain; this only leads to involuntary tensing of the muscles, the opposite of the intended effect. Sometimes, temporarily slowing

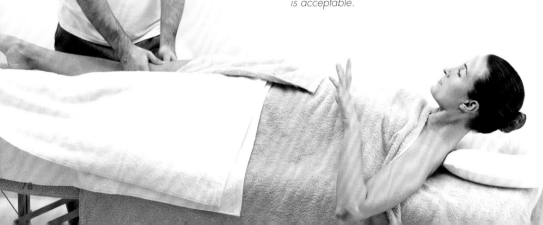

Checking the pressure
Be sure to ask at regular intervals if the pressure of your massage is acceptable.

or lessening pressure will allow the receiver to adjust to the sensations sufficiently to allow you to resume without further problem. Otherwise, it may be advisable to move on to the next area to be treated.

Calling a halt

There are some rare situations in which it may be advisable to end the session before it is complete. Discontinue the massage if the receiver:

- Requests you to stop, for whatever reason.
- Complains of faintness or loses consciousness.
- Behaves inappropriately toward you.

Is Everything OK?

At each stage of the massage, from getting changed to the point at which the person leaves, be sure to inquire gently whether the person is happy with what is happening. For example, you might ask: Are you warm enough? Is the position comfortable? Would you like a drink of water? Use your instinct and common sense to respond to the person's needs.

When the Massage Has Finished

When you have completed the massage, use a clean towel to wipe excess oil from the back and make sure there is a towel for the person to wipe other parts of the body as needed before they get dressed. In most amateur situations you won't be able to offer a shower, but if one is available, this is ideal.

It is important to allow the person some minutes to relax after the massage and absorb the benefits of the treatment. Make sure they are warm enough and provide an extra cover if required. Offer a glass of water, as massage can leave the receiver thirsty. Leave the room so that the person can relax and then get dressed. Remember to knock before returning.

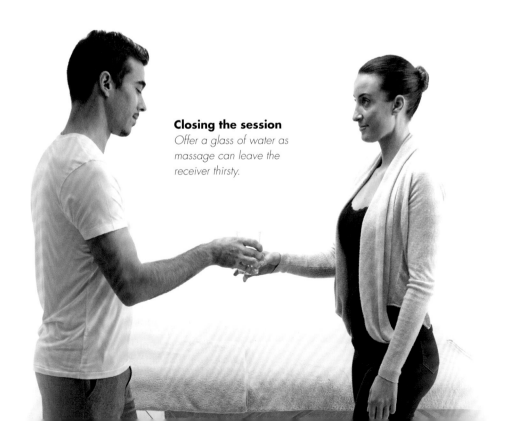

Closing the session
Offer a glass of water as massage can leave the receiver thirsty.

Before leaving

Once the person is dressed, be sure to inquire how they are feeling. Massage is intended to be relaxing so tell them that it may not be advisable to drive or cycle until they are fully alert. You should also make the person aware of the normal possible physiological after-effects of massage treatment. Explain that these are signs that the treatment has had a positive effect on the body and are not a cause for concern. These may last for a few hours and may include:

- Aching muscles.
- Increased urination.
- Increased bowel activity.
- Slight headache (a severe headache should not be assumed to be the result of massage).
- Increased thirst.
- Drowsiness.
- Temporary sleep disturbance.

After-massage advice

It is important to tell anyone who has received massage to do the following in the 12 hours after the treatment:

- Drink plenty of water.
- Take a warm shower or bath.
- Avoid alcohol or other stimulants.
- Eat only light meals.
- Rest.

BASIC
TECHNIQUES

You now have an understanding of the tradition and theories that underlie massage therapy, and have learned how to prepare yourself and your environment. In this chapter you will be introduced to the essential techniques of massage, from the use of oils to the basic considerations of direction and pressure of the strokes. Clear explanations of each of the main massage strokes are accompanied by helpful illustrations to provide you with the skills you need to embark on your practice.

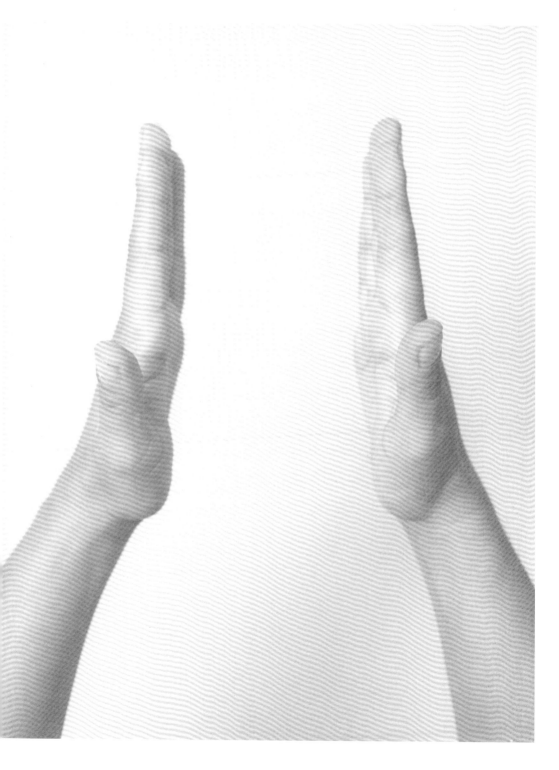

Lubricant Oils & Massage

Massage involves the direct contact and movement of your hands over the receiver's bare skin. In most cases, some form of lubricating massage medium is needed to reduce the amount of friction between the skin surfaces, which could create soreness and discomfort. However, you need to use careful judgment based on your knowledge and information arising from your initial conversation with the person receiving the massage to decide which oil is most appropriate to use. You will also need to give thought to whether you want to add one or more essential oils to the basic (or carrier) oil to add the benefits of aromatherapy to your practice. More detail about the use of essential oils is given later in this section.

A basic oil

You do not need to invest in expensive or rare oils for most massage, but it is important to choose an oil that carries the least risk of provoking an allergic reaction. One of the best general-purpose oils is sunflower oil. Choose a high-quality product that is both cold-pressed and organic. Other oils that may be used

have potential disadvantages and are probably best avoided unless there is a good reason for their use. In particular, it is best to avoid oils derived from nuts unless you are absolutely certain that they are safe, because of the risk of a reaction if the person has a nut allergy. Overleaf you will find details about some of the most popular options.

Applying oil for massage

Having chosen your oil, you'll need to know how and when to apply it. A key consideration is temperature. The sudden shock of cold liquid on the skin can provoke immediate tensing of the muscles—the last thing you need at the start of a massage. Always dispense a small amount of oil into the palm of one hand and then rub your hands together to distribute it evenly across both palms. This also ensures that you do not use too much, which could lead to the skin becoming too slippery. Repeat the process whenever you sense that the skin is becoming too dry for your hands to move smoothly over the surface.

Avoiding Allergic Reactions

Your introductory conversation with the person you are about to massage should always include a question about known allergies, and this will guide your choice of oils. But the person may not be aware of their potential to have a reaction to all substances, so it is wise to be cautious. Only use the least allergenic of oils and essential oils until you are sure other substances are safe. To check this, you will need to perform a patch test 48 hours before the treatment—apply the proposed oil to a small area (1 sq cm) of skin. Advise the person to avoid washing the area and check for redness or irritation when they return for the massage. If the skin is unaffected, you can safely use the oil.

Always advise against a sauna or hot bath immediately before massage, as this increases the likelihood of a skin reaction to the oil.

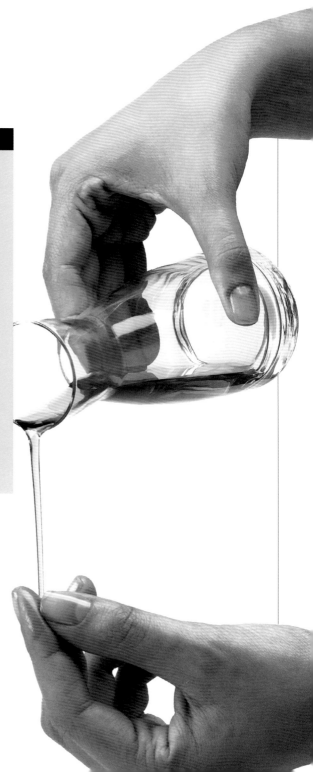

WHICH LUBRICANT OIL? Choose a high-quality product that is both cold-pressed and organic. Sunflower oil is the best all-purpose oil. Some of the oils listed here have potential disadvantages and are probably best avoided unless there is a good reason for their use.

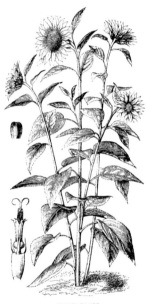

SUNFLOWER

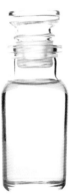

GRAPESEED

Sunflower (*Helianthus annuus*)
- Rich in vitamins A, D, E and in calcium, zinc, iron, potassium, and phosphorus.
- Very good general-purpose oil for full-body massage.

Grapeseed (*Vitus vinifera*)
- Finely textured, not sticky or viscous. Nourishes and protects the skin. High in linoleic acid, a polyunsaturated fatty acid. Contains traces of vitamin E, which adds to the keeping properties of the oil.
- Good for body massage, but may cause staining of towels and clothing.

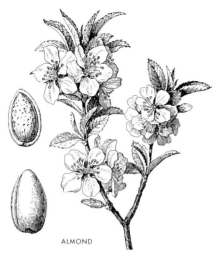

ALMOND

Sweet almond oil (*Prunus amygdalus* var. *dulcus*)

- Oily texture provides effective lubrication, but has the potential to cause allergic reactions in individuals who have a nut allergy.
- A good massage oil that should be used only after a patch test.

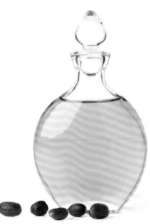

JOJOBA

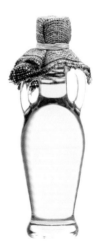

OLIVE OIL

Jojoba (*Simmondsia chinensis*)

- Finely textured, not sticky, and readily absorbed. Its chemical structure is similar to that of sebum, the skin's natural oil. Its ability to dissolve sebum makes it useful for clearing the pores in acne-prone skin. Contains myristic acid, an anti-inflammatory agent, therefore can be of benefit for arthritis and rheumatism.
- A good choice for all kinds of massage.

Olive oil (*Olea europaea*)

- Calming, soothing, and emollient. Aids healing of burns, bruises, and sprains. Said to relieve insect bites and itchy skin, and is both mildly astringent and antiseptic.
- May be too thick and sticky for full-body massage.

Essential Oils & Massage

Natural fragrance

Essential oils extracted from plants and added to a lubricant oil can enhance the benefits of massage.

Our sense of smell is linked to an area that is often seen as the most primitive part of the brain, the limbic system. As well as registering the smells we encounter, it also controls functions such as mood and memory. Most people have experienced being cast back to an early experience by a familiar scent, whether baking bread evoking the kitchen of their childhood or the smell of the sea bringing back happy memories of family holidays. As a practitioner of massage, you can use the power of smell to enhance your practice by adding essential oils to your basic massage oil.

Using aromatherapy

Aromatherapy is a complex natural remedy system that involves the use of highly concentrated essences—essential oils—of aromatic plants to produce emotional and physical benefits. Aromatherapists ascribe specific healing benefits to each essential oil. The oils are either inhaled as vapor or diluted in a carrier oil and applied to the skin.

You do not need to be a fully qualified aromatherapist to utilize the insights of the system for the benefit of the people to whom you give massage, and with a few notable exceptions the oils are entirely safe for use on the skin.

Most people enjoy spending time in a fragrant room and are happy to have pleasantly scented oils applied to their skin, but it is always wise to check with the person that they are happy for you to incorporate essential oils into your treatment. And importantly, avoid the use of essential oils on pregnant women.

WHICH ESSENTIAL OIL?

The oils described below are all safe to add to a basic massage (carrier) oil in the proportions recommended. Most of the time you will probably want to select one or more essential oils that are generally relaxing, but as you become more experienced you may decide to try oils that may bring more specific healing benefits. Ready blended oils are available, but these restrict your ability to adapt the blend to suit individual needs.

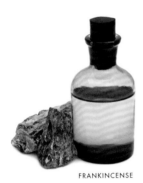

FRANKINCENSE

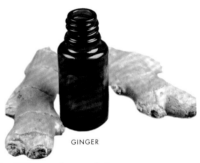

GINGER

Selected essential oils for massage

The following list is a small selection of the many essential oils available. You can add your own favorites to your practice, but be sure to check a reputable reference resource for possible risks and side effects before using them in massage oil.

Benzoin (*Styrax benzoin*)
- Warming, relaxing. Good for respiratory conditions, circulatory problems, aching muscles and joints.
- Risk of reaction in sensitive skin.

Frankincense (*Boswellia carteri*)
- Relaxing, warming, mood-lifting.

Geranium (*Pelargonium graveleons*)
- Pain-relieving, anti-inflammatory, cooling, relaxing, mood-lifting. Good for oily skin.

Ginger (*Zingiber officinale*)
- Stimulating, warming, wakes up the body.
- Avoid using on sensitive skin. Risk of skin irritation. Use no more than 4 drops per 20 ml of carrier oil.

How Much Oil to Use

For a healthy adult, use a maximum of 8 drops of essential oil to 20 ml of carrier oil (this is usually the right amount for a full-body massage). For a face massage, 2 drops of essential oil in 5 ml of carrier oil is sufficient. Halve the amount of essential oil for children and frail or elderly people. It is advisable to use a maximum of three different essential oils in a single blend.

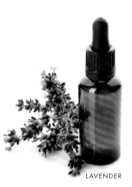

LAVENDER

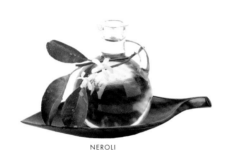

NEROLI

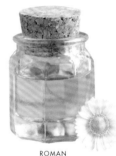

ROMAN
CHAMOMILE

Grapefruit (*Citrus paradis*)

- Astringent, purifying, fungicidal, stimulating, mood-lifting.
- Grapefruit is generally safe but it can cause irritation if, following application, the skin is exposed to sunlight. Be sure to warn about this possible side effect.

Lavender (*Lavandula angustifolia*)

- Analgesic, anti-inflammatory, antispasmodic, antiseptic, fungicidal, balancing, cooling, relaxing, mood-lifting.
- Lavender is neither toxic nor irritant—one of the most useful essential oils for massage and room fragrance.

Neroli (*Citrus aurantium* var. *amara*)

- Counters anxiety, stress, and emotional upsets, sedative, relaxing.

Palmarosa (*Cymbopogon martini*)

- Antibacterial, antifungal, calming, promotes healthy heart function, hydrating, sedative.

Roman chamomile (*Chamaemelum nobile*)

- Pain-relieving, anti-inflammatory, antispasmodic, antiseptic, antiviral.

Sandalwood (*Santalum album*)

- Pain-relieving, antidepressant, antiseptic, promotes cell renewal, stimulating, restorative. Good for aching muscles.

Essential Principles

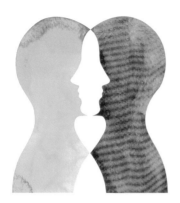

Self-awareness
*To provide effective massage,
keep the essential principles
in mind as you work.*

Before you start your massage practice, it is important to understand and incorporate into your approach the essential principles that underpin all good massage. These are often called the Four Gems. Using these principles to guide your hands and mind when you are giving massage provides a sound basis for the success of the treatment.

The Four Gems

The idea of the Four Gems has its origins in Buddhist teachings that refer to four divine states of mind: metta (selflessness), karuna (understanding), mudita (joy for others), and uppekha (openness to others). The Four Gems of massage—Intention, Focus, Rhythm, and Continuity—have some parallels with these qualities. The internalizing of this underlying philosophy, and the way you build its principles into your practice, will give the massage you offer the ability to provide restorative healing to the people you treat.

Intention

This refers to your underlying purpose in giving the massage. To be effective, a serious masseur needs to have a complete commitment to providing, through their hands, a healing touch—a kind of selflessness. Before and during the treatment, keep in mind that your intention is to benefit the well-being of the receiver. All personal concerns must be set aside. This attitude will inform your conversations with the person you are treating and will also be conveyed through your hands while the massage is in progress.

Focus

The ability to exclude irrelevant considerations and personal feelings

is key to the detachment necessary to
provide the best possible massage.
Having focus allows you to maintain the
intention of the massage at the forefront
of your mind. The centering techniques
discussed on pages 56–57 can help you
prevent your mind drifting toward outside
distractions and concerns.

Focus also refers to how you align
your gaze during massage. Always
keep your gaze focused on the area you
are massaging to enable you to notice
changes as you work.

Rhythm

The human body responds to harmony and rhythm through the ears, as in our appreciation of music, and through the eyes when we respond to visual art. In the same way, the sense of touch reacts positively to harmonious contact from another person. Massage strokes that are given rhythmically and confidently elicit relaxation and bodily cooperation from the receiver, whereas, conversely, hesitant and erratic contact creates tension and resistance.

Rhythm should not only be present in your physical contact with the receiver, but also throughout the consultation.

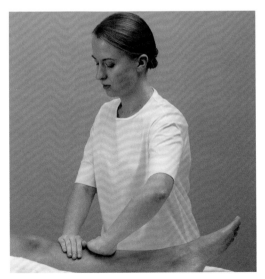

Learn to keep in mind the need to gently guide the person you are treating through the different phases from initial conversation and preparation through changes of position during the massage and ending the treatment, without interruption and with a reassuring flow.

Continuity

This gem is connected to rhythm but also takes in a further aspect to good massage practice. One of the most important practical techniques, to the extent that it might even be considered a rule, is to maintain physical contact with the person throughout the massage if at all possible. In the following pages you will learn about the importance of establishing a grounding contact at the start of the massage. Having made this initial positive connection, you should try not to break it. Learn to keep at least one hand in contact with the receiver's body as you change position.

Inner focus
*Maintain contact
and focus throught
the massage treatment.*

Direction & pressure

These considerations are additional to the Four Gems, but are nevertheless fundamental to massage practice and are an important part of what makes classic massage different from the touch of untrained hands. Think of a typical effleurage (see page 98) massage stroke like the movement of waves on a shore. The forward movement of the stroke is like the waves breaking, strong and forward moving. The return movement is gentler, like the ebb of the water.

Direction

When applying massage strokes, it is important to consider the direction of the forward movement. Usually you will need to work toward the heart—that is, the center of the body. In other words, apply the stroke from the extremities toward the torso.

Pressure

The amount of force you apply to each stroke is critical in obtaining the desired benefit of the massage. Use too much pressure and you risk causing pain, which will in turn lead to unwanted

tensing of the muscles. And too light a stroke will fail to provide sufficient stimulation of the muscle and therefore be ineffective, and in some cases might be felt as tickling rather than as relaxing contact. The trick is to achieve a balance.

As a general rule, first ask the person if they have had massage before and whether they prefer a strong or light touch. It is best to start with a fairly light pressure to accustom the person to the contact. You can gradually increase the pressure you use as you repeat the strokes. Always ask the person repeatedly during the course of the massage if the pressure feels right to them.

Effleurage

The classic gliding stroke of massage, effleurage is the introductory stroke for almost all massages. The term derives from the French word *effleurer*, which means to skim or touch lightly. It is used to introduce the receiver to the touch of the person giving the massage and as a soothing end-of-massage stroke. It is also the stroke you use for distributing massage oil over the skin in the area to be massaged.

What are the benefits?

Effleurage stimulates the circulation, warms and relaxes the muscles, and aids the removal of toxins from the tissues via the lymphatic system and bloodstream. It also releases and removes dead skin cells from the skin surface, clearing the pores and aiding the flow of sebum.

What to do

Effleurage utilizes the flat of the hands and involves both the palms and fingers. The fingers and thumbs should always be closed, with no gaps between them.

Place both hands on the skin—either side by side for larger areas, or one ahead of the other, aligned in opposite directions on narrower parts of the body, such as the calves.

This is your first physical contact with the person, so pause for a few moments to allow them to adjust to your touch. Breathe deeply and evenly and use this pause to focus on the treatment to come and allow your confident contact to instill trust in the receiver.

Keeping the whole hand (palm and fingers) in contact with the skin, move the hands over the skin in the direction of the heart. Although initially effleurage should not involve heavy pressure, it should carry sufficient weight to create a positive contact. The stroke then returns, with a lighter pressure, to the starting point. The aim is to create a gentle rhythm with gradually increasing pressure. Be sure to generate the movement with your whole body, not just the arms and shoulders, transferring your weight forward from your back leg onto the front leg.

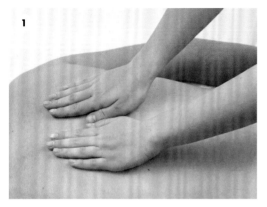

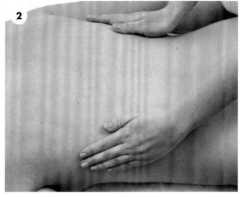

Effleurage for larger areas

1 *Using the flat of both hands, apply medium pressure in the direction of the heart.*

2 *Maintaining contact with a lighter pressure, bring both hands back to the starting position.*

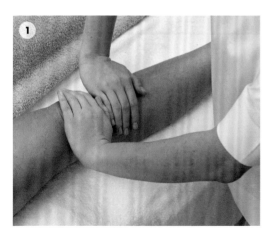

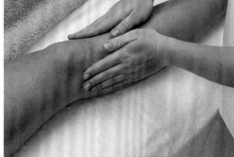

Effleurage for smaller areas

1 *For narrow areas of the body, such as the arms and legs, use both hands angled in opposite directions for the initial stroke.*

2 *For the lighter return sroke, place the hands on either side of the arm or leg.*

Petrissage

Following the introduction of contact through effleurage, the classic order of massage involves the application of strokes of medium pressure. This group of strokes comes under the general heading "petrissage." The French word *pétrir*, from which petrissage derives, means to knead, as when making bread. But kneading is only one of several petrissage strokes. Petrissage is used when muscles have become stiff and tense as a result of excessive use or emotional stress. These strokes stretch the muscle fibers and boost circulation to the tissues, which helps the removal of toxins.

Kneading

This massage technique uses a lifting and squeezing action of both hands to free tension in large muscles. This vigorous stroke increases muscle elasticity and permits the muscles to relax. But the firmness of the contact can also be stimulating and energizing.

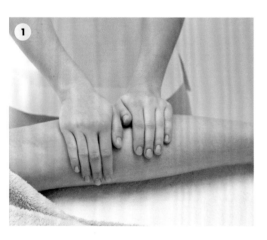

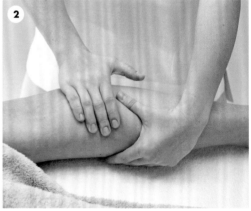

Kneading
1 *Place both hands side by side.*

2,3 *Use the thumb of one hand to push forwards and the fingers of the other hand to pull back to lift the flesh away from the bone, then reverse the action.*

What to do

Use kneading on areas where there are muscles with sufficient bulk to be grasped in the hand. It cannot be applied to areas where the muscles are thin and close to the bone. Use your whole body to create the rhythm and apply the necessary pressure.

Use both hands side by side to grasp the flesh.

With the thumb of one hand and the fingers of the other, lift the flesh away from the bone, then reverse the action.

Alternate this action in a flowing and rhythmic movement that replicates a kneading action.

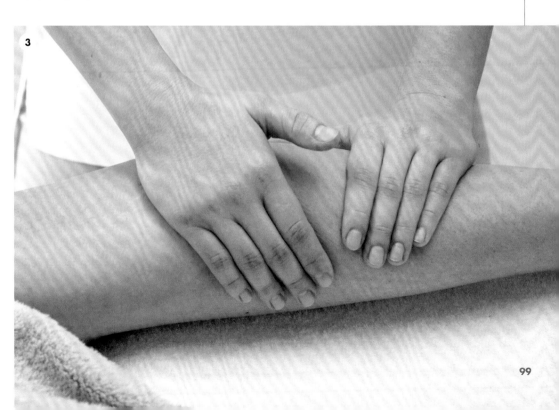

3

99

Wringing

Typically used on a limb, this stroke has similar benefits to kneading. It stretches and releases tension in the muscles. When using this stroke, begin conservatively, applying only a moderate amount of pressure. Only increase the squeeze when you are sure the person you are treating can tolerate it.

What to do

Cup your hands over the limb. Keeping fingers and thumbs together and the palms and fingers in contact with the skin, move one hand forward and the other one back to squeeze the muscle underneath. Then rhythmically reverse the action. Gradually move the hands along the limb to work the whole muscle.

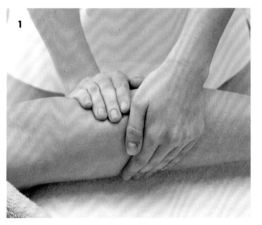 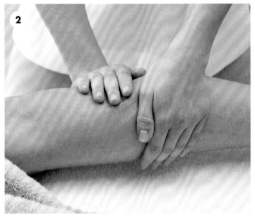

Wringing
1, 2 Move one hand forward and the other back to squeeze the muscle. Then reverse the action.

Double-handed caterpillar squeeze

This petrissage technique can be used to squeeze and soften the larger muscles of limbs.

What to do

Place both hands side by side over the area to be treated. Grasp the muscle with both hands and lift it firmly away from the bone.

Move the hands along the limb and repeat to treat the whole muscle.

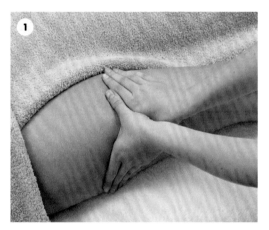 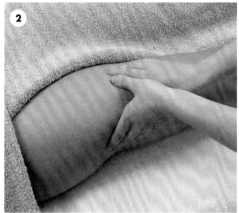

Double-handed caterpillar squeeze
1, 2 *With both hands side by side but with the fingers in opposite directions, grasp the muscle and lift it firmly away from the bone. Repeat the action as you move along the limb.*

One-handed caterpillar squeeze

This technique is used to stimulate the smaller muscles, particularly of the arms and legs.

What to do

Use one hand to lift and squeeze the muscle. Quickly release and continue to alternate this rapid plucking action, moving along the area under treatment.

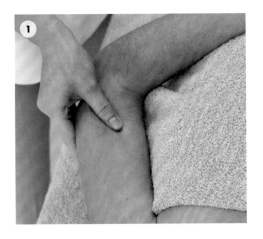 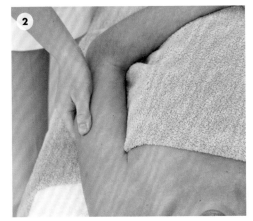

One-handed caterpillar squeeze

1, 2 *Use the thumb and the fingers to grasp a portion of flesh and gently pull it upward. Release and repeat as you move up the limb. Use the static hand to provide continuous contact nearby.*

Applying deeper pressure

Strokes of this type are mainly used to dispel tension and knots deep within muscles. In most cases, these strokes involve focused pressure from the thumbs and/or fingers, often applied in a circling motion. In some cases, it may be appropriate to use the heel of the hand or even the elbow to apply pressure.

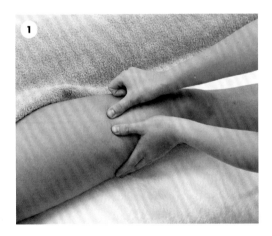

Thumb pressure
1 *Use both thumbs to apply gradually increasing pressure. As you do so, make small circling movements. Release and move the thumbs to the next position to be worked and repeat.*

What to do

Use both hands together. Place the pads of the thumbs over the area to be worked, while gently enclosing the area with your fingers and hands. You can use finger pressure in very much the same way as for thumb pressure.

Use the weight of your body to apply gradually increasing pressure to the area. Breathe slowly and deeply throughout the process.

As you increase the pressure, make small circling movements with your thumbs, feeling the gradual freeing of the tissues beneath. You will soon sense when the area has been worked sufficiently (increasing warmth is a good indicator), but while you are learning, work each area for a maximum count of ten before moving on to the next section of the area under treatment. Avoid working an area for longer as this may cause soreness. The application of pressure for too long may also temporarily block the circulation of blood to the muscle. Apply a few effleurage strokes after each application of thumb pressure to restore blood flow.

Percussion Strokes

I n contrast to the relaxing, gliding strokes of effleurage and the stretching, squeezing and releasing effects of petrissage, percussion strokes (sometimes called tapotement) are intended to tone and stimulate the muscles, and are most often used toward the end of a massage. Most of these brisk and rapid strokes should not be used on areas where the bone is close to the skin, such as the shins or spine. Percussion strokes include hacking, pounding, cupping, and plucking. The "raindrop" technique, which involves gentle tapping, is a further stroke within this category, and can be used on more delicate areas.

"Raindrop" Technique

Although not needed for any of the massages in this book, the "raindrop" stroke is a gentle tapping action that can be used to treat delicate areas where the bone is close to the surface, such as the face and neck. The effect is both relaxing and gently stimulating.

With hands and fingers relaxed, use the fingertips to tap the area, using a fluttering action. Keep the action light and "bouncy." This stroke involves very little pressure.

Hacking

This stroke uses the outer edge of the hand to apply brisk, chopping strokes to the area under treatment.

What to do

With elbows bent and arms relaxed, hold both hands, palms facing and fingers open, over the area. Throughout the process, keep your wrists relaxed and flexible.

Using a rapid up and down action, strike the muscle with each hand alternately. As one hand makes contact, immediately lift it and strike with the other. The force should not be too great, and the movement should be brisk and rhythmic. Gradually increase the force of the stroke according to the needs and tolerance of the receiver.

Be sure to work over the whole muscle evenly and be careful not to spend too much time working any one area. This might cause soreness.

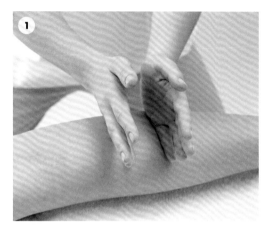

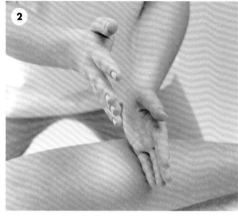

Hacking

1 *Place both hands over the area to be treated, thumbs uppermost and with palms facing.*

2 *Using the hands alternately, make contact with the area to be treated with the edge of the hand in a chopping action.*

3 *Continue in a brisk rhythm, moving along the whole area under treatment.*

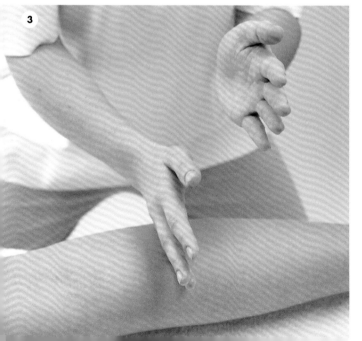

105

Pounding

This type of percussion stroke utilizes the fists to apply pressure in much the same way as in hacking. It should be used only on well-muscled areas.

What to do

Form your hands into loose fists (do not clench the fists tightly) and hold them, little finger side downward, over the muscle to be treated. Hold your elbows outward and have your fists close together.

Using the hands alternately, pound the muscle with a bouncy rhythm. Start slowly with light pressure and build up speed and force as appropriate.

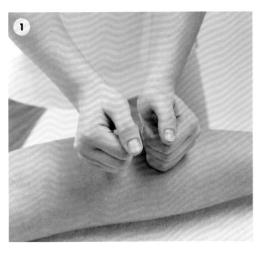 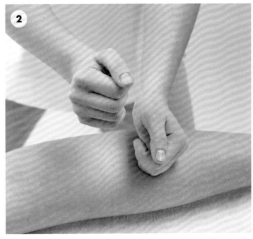

Pounding
1, 2 *Use the outside edge of your fists alternately to pound the area under treatment.*

Cupping

This stroke consists of a percussive action that creates a momentary vacuum between the hand and the recipient's skin and is particularly stimulating to the circulation. For this reason, it may cause warming and reddening of the skin during treatment.

What to do

With fingers and thumbs together, form a cup with both hands. Place them palm down over the area to be treated.

Alternately raise and lower each hand onto the area under treatment with a brisk and rhythmic action. A clapping sound is created when each hand makes contact with the skin.

As you raise each hand, reform it into a cupped shape ready for the next stroke.

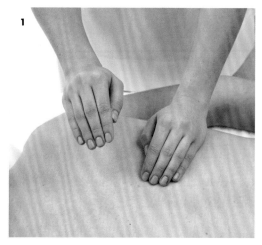
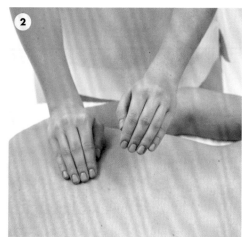

Cupping
1, 2 Form a cup shape with each hand. Firmly tap the area with each hand alternately in a rhythmic action.

Additional Massage Techniques

There are several massage techniques in addition to the classic massage strokes that can form part of the massage therapist's armory. In many cases, these derive from massage traditions from around the world and have centuries of practice to validate their effectiveness. While these are not always included in the massage sequences later in this book, once you have gained experience and confidence you may wish to incorporate them in your practice.

Vibration

This is a technique commonly used to dispel tension and stiffness in tight muscles, particularly where petrissage treatment has not been successful.

What to do

Place the whole hand (for a large muscle) or just the fingertips (for smaller areas) over the area to be treated. Using firm pressure, rapidly move the hand (or fingertips) from side to side to agitate the muscle below, moving the muscle but without sliding the hand (or fingertips) over the skin. You can stabilize the hand by placing the other hand on top.

Static pressure

Shiatsu treatment involves exerting pressure on specific points in the body to improve the flow of energy. However, you do not have to subscribe to the ideas behind shiatsu to utilize some of its techniques. Thumb and finger pressure are used in some of the massages in this book, and you can take this approach further by using other parts of your body to apply pressure to release deep-seated tension.

What to do

To apply deep pressure to tissues below large muscles such as those on the

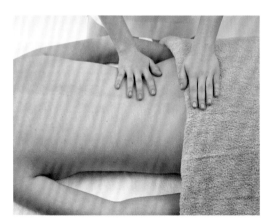

Vibration
The muscles of the back, thighs or legs are effectively relaxed by the use of vibration.

buttocks around the hip, you can use the heel of your hand or even your elbow.

When using the heel of your hand, stabilize the area being worked with the flat of one hand, while placing the heel of the working hand directly over the area in which you wish to apply pressure.

Keeping the arm straight, use your weight to apply pressure through the heel of the hand. Hold for a few seconds, release, and repeat in a rhythmic sequence.

Follow a similar method of working when using the elbow. Be sure not to exert too much pressure or to maintain the pressure for too long.

Joint mobilization

Practitioners of massage often utilize passive joint movements to improve mobility of the limbs.

What to do

This involves the practitioner gently moving the joint (for example, hip, shoulder, or ankle) through its full range of movement. This is usually done following the application of massage strokes to relax the surrounding muscles. The recipient needs to release conscious control of the joint and allow you to control the movement.

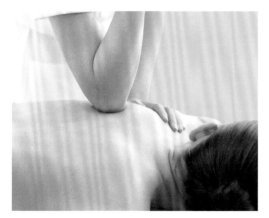

Static pressure
The elbow can be used to apply pressure on large muscles.

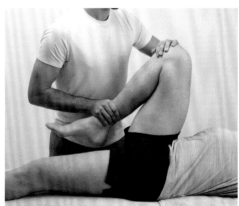

Joint mobilization
Moving a joint such as the hip through its full range of movement improves mobility.

Finishing Techniques

When you have completed your massage treatment, whether you have worked on the whole body or only a part of it, it is vital to end the session in a way that integrates and prolongs the benefits. The usual way is to use long effleurage strokes to link the areas that have been treated. Just as when starting a massage (see page 96), gently but firmly glide your hands in a circular pattern over the body in the direction of the heart.

The end of massage effleurage need not be as long as the introductory phase, and should be relatively gentle.

Closure

When you have completed the effleurage at the end of your massage session, keep your hands in place on the receiver's body and focus on the treatment you have given for a few moments. Breathe deeply and calmly and focus on transferring this peaceful and healing energy to the person you have been treating.

Finally, cover the person with towels and let them know that the massage has finished.

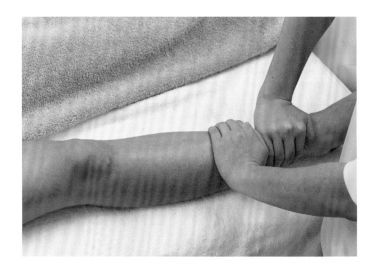

Closing effleurage
End your massage with flowing efleurage strokes over the area or areas that have been treated.

FULL-BODY
MASSAGE ROUTINE

Massage of the whole body not only provides a restorative general treatment for the person receiving the massage, but also allows the giver of the massage the opportunity to practice a wide variety of strokes and techniques. This chapter describes a standard routine for a full-body massage in segments divided by area of the body. The anatomical features of each part are described, along with step-by-step instructions on the strokes to use on that area. By following these instructions, you will have the information you need to provide an effective general-purpose massage.

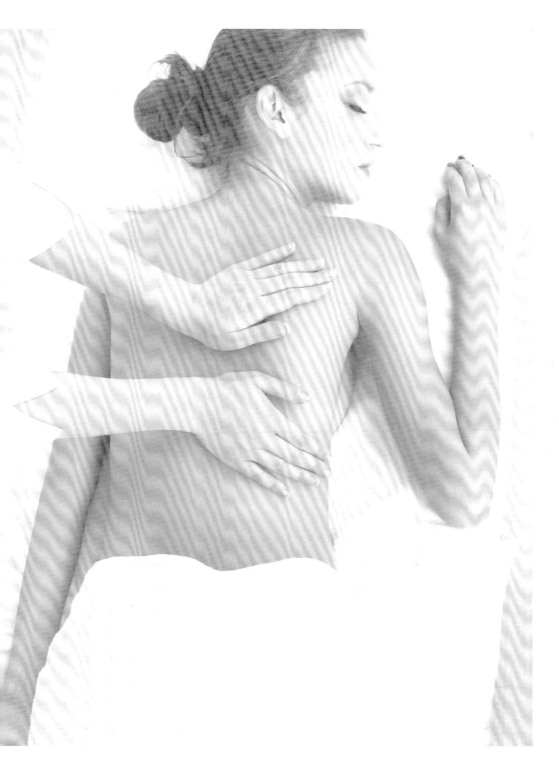

Full-Body Massage Essentials

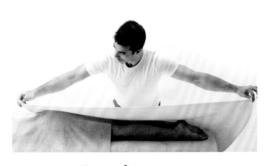

A complete process

A full-body massage allows the therapist to put into practice a wide range of skills and techniques.

Massage that treats most areas of the body is the mainstay of massage practice. Unless the aim is to focus on a specific problem area or time is short, treating the whole body is the preferred option. It allows the therapist to investigate and address areas of tension that may not have been apparent to the person being treated or that have arisen as a consequence of problems elsewhere in the body. It can be seen as the equivalent of a full service for your car.

Many people enjoy a regular full-body massage as part of a strategy for health maintenance, in the same way as they might build in regular visits to the gym or take vitamin supplements. Regular receivers of this form of therapy report that it helps to dispel the harmful effects of stress, and keeps at bay many chronic health problems, such as backache and recurrent headaches.

A learning process

Learning to give a full-body massage has many benefits for a novice practitioner. It enables you to utilize almost every massage technique, from applying the different strokes to the way you put into practice the philosophy of massage as expressed in the Four Gems. You will learn to maneuver yourself and the person receiving the massage into the correct position at each stage. Moving from one part of the body to the next means that you have to consider the vital principles of rhythm and continuity. And at the same time you will be practicing the consideration and care that are essential qualities for a good massage technique.

A full-body massage is unlikely to be the first massage project you undertake. It requires considerable concentration and focus, which can sometimes take time to acquire. You may wish to practice

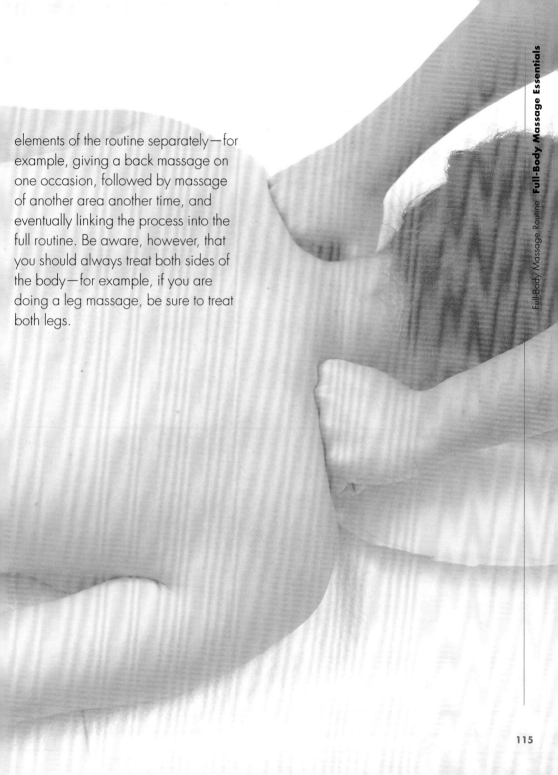

elements of the routine separately—for example, giving a back massage on one occasion, followed by massage of another area another time, and eventually linking the process into the full routine. Be aware, however, that you should always treat both sides of the body—for example, if you are doing a leg massage, be sure to treat both legs.

Selection of strokes

The routine on the following pages includes a full program of relaxing and stimulating strokes that will provide an effective massage for most people. However, it is important to use your judgment based on the special needs of the individual you are treating. In particular, you may wish to limit your use of percussion strokes if you do not want to stimulate the area and your aim is to create an overall effect of relaxation.

Timing

A full-body massage cannot be hurried. You need to allow sufficient time to complete the massage without rushing the final stages, which are as important as the first part of the routine. And while you are working you may discover areas that require more attention than you predicted. There can be no absolute guidelines for how long the routine will take, but it may be advisable to warn the person to allow a minimum two hours, which would include a preliminary conversation and after-massage chat.

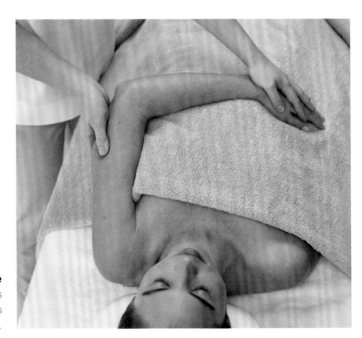

Taking time
During a full-body massage, always allow yourself time to focus on areas that need extra attention.

Full-Body Massage Checklist

- Before you start the massage, it's a good idea to run through a checklist of the essential preparations that were discussed in more detail in Part 3.

- Is the room ready? In particular, check the temperature and cleanliness.

- Do you have all you need to hand? Check there are sufficient clean towels to cover the table and to drape the person you are treating. Make sure you have sufficient massage oil. If adding essential oils, prepare the blend in advance, where possible.

- Are you ready? Be sure to be physically comfortable and mentally focused at the start.

- Remember to apply oil to each area of the body before you start massaging it.

Phase 1 • Face Down

A full-body massage normally starts with the receiver lying face down on the massage table. Before you start, be sure that the person you are treating is comfortable and completely draped with two large towels. Gently check that they are lying as symmetrically as possible, carefully adjusting their position as necessary. If you have a massage table with a hole for the face, make sure their face is comfortably positioned over the hole and the neck is straight. If you are using a massage table without a hole, support the forehead with a folded towel.

Initial grounding

1 Stand with your feet slightly apart. With the towel still in place, rest your hands, fingers together, on the middle of the back. Focus on the contact while taking three breaths.

Direction & order

The face-down phase starts with the lower legs and moves up the body to finish with a scalp massage.

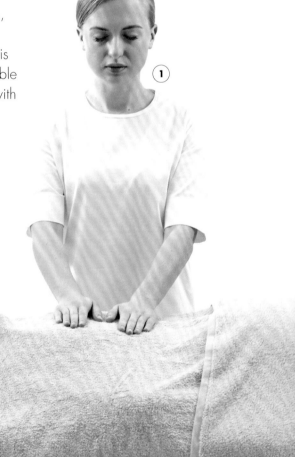

Grounding

Before you start massage of any part of the body, it is important to begin with a grounding touch. This introduces the receiver to contact with your hands before any actual massage takes place.

First moves
2 *Turn to face the head and gently move both hands down the thigh toward the calf, using an effleurage stroke.*

Grounding on the calf
3 *Move to stand beside the calf and place your hands on the calf, towel in place, for a further count of three.*

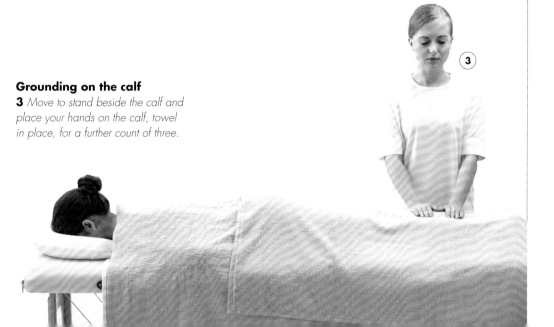

BACK OF CALF

The calf (or back of the lower leg) is the area between the ankle and the back of the knee. For the massage therapist, the most important feature of this part of the body is the large muscle known as the gastrocnemius (see page 31). This muscle, familiarly known as the calf muscle, is formed of two sections on either side of the back of the lower leg. It is joined by a tendon (Achilles tendon) to the ankle bones and to the bones above the knee. This is a hardworking muscle that contracts every time we flex our feet. It can become tense through overuse and also is shortened in those who, over the years, have frequently worn high heels. Massage of this muscle can help to ease stiffness and improve flexibility and ease of movement.

Treat Both Sides

When you have completed treatment of the calf, the thigh, and the whole leg on one side, move to the other side of the table and treat the other leg in the same way before moving on to the next segment.

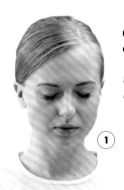

Grounding on the calf
1 *Fold back the towel from one calf and rest both hands on the calf.*

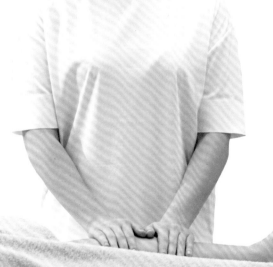

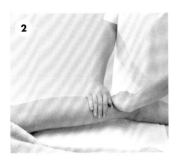

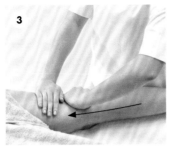

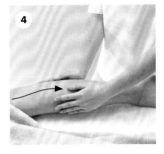

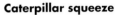

Initial effleurage
2, 3 *Turn to face the head. Place both hands above the ankle and apply an effleurage stroke up the calf toward the knee.*

Completing the stroke
4 *Bring the hands back toward the ankle down the sides of the calf. Repeat steps 2–4 three times.*

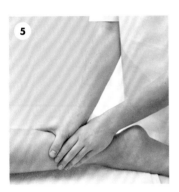

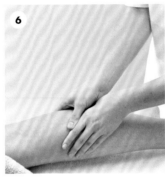

Caterpillar squeeze
5, 6 *Apply a double-handed caterpillar squeeze and lift up the fleshy part of the calf. Repeat three times.*

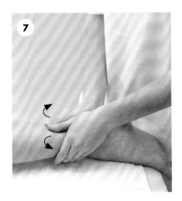

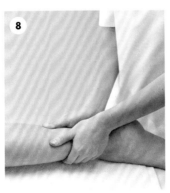

Thumb pressure
7, 8 *Apply pressure with both thumbs in a circular motion all the way up the calf, moving from the ankle to just below the knee. Treat the whole calf by working in three lines: middle, outer, and inner calf.*

Continued overleaf

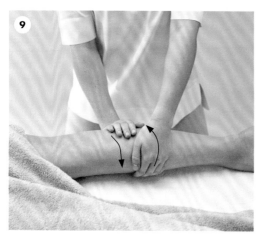

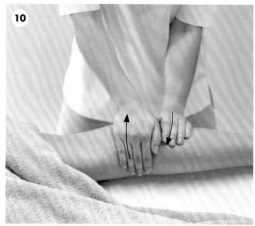

Wringing
9, 10 *Use a wringing technique to alternately push and pull the calf muscle.*

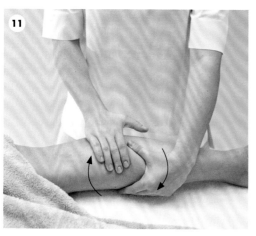

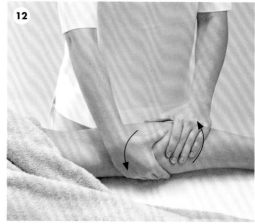

Kneading
11, 12 *Using both hands in an alternating movement, lift and squeeze the calf muscle along its length.*

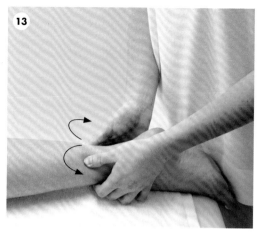

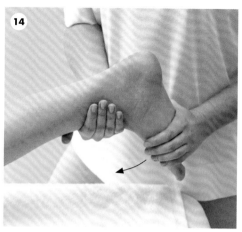

Thumb pressure on the Achilles tendon
13 *Use the thumbs to apply pressure in a circling motion over the Achilles, above the back of the ankle.*

Stretching the calf muscles
14 *Place one hand under the ankle and push down the foot with your other hand. Hold for three seconds and release. Repeat three times.*

Calf shake
15 *Hold the foot in both hands and shake with a small movement.*

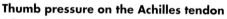

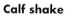

123

BACK OF THE THIGH

The main muscles at the back of the thigh, popularly known as the hamstrings, extend from the pelvis to the knee. When these muscles contract, the leg bends at the knee—a movement that most of us perform innumerable times every day. The muscles at the back of the thigh can become tense and stiff after unusual exercise, and are often shortened in those who spend much of the day sitting in a chair. Massage can help to counteract these problems, which can potentially adversely affect posture and mobility. Each of the strokes in this segment should be followed by a linking effleurage stroke.

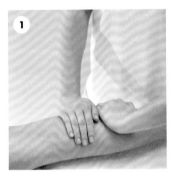

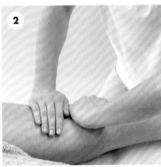

Effleurage

1, 2 *Fold the towel back to reveal the back of the thigh. Apply an effleurage stroke from the calf to the top of the thigh. Start with light pressure and gradually increase the pressure as you repeat the stroke three times.*

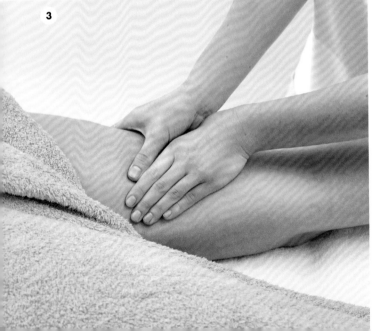

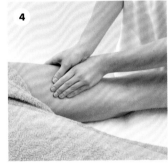

Caterpillar squeeze

3, 4 *Apply caterpillar squeezes with both hands to grasp and lift the muscle at the back of the thigh. Work from the knee to the top of the thigh.*

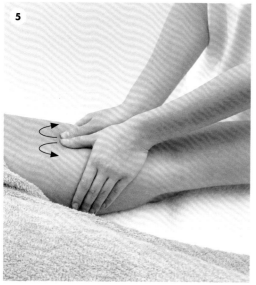

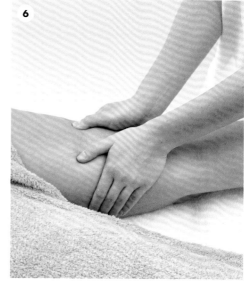

Thumb pressure

5, 6 *Appy circling thumb pressure up the back of the thigh.*
Work in three strips: up the middle, inside, and outside of the thigh.

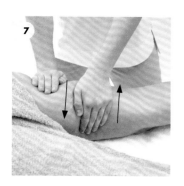

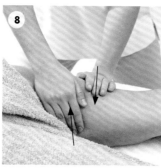

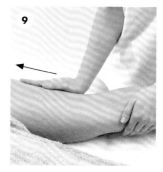

Wringing

7, 8 *Use both hands working in opposite directions across the back of the thigh to apply a wringing stroke to the muscle.*

Heel of hand

9 *Use the heel of one hand to apply smooth pressure up the outside of the thigh. Circle back and repeat three times.*

WHOLE LEG

Having worked to loosen the lower and upper parts of the leg separately, you need to apply some linking strokes to integrate the benefits. First use percussion strokes to stimulate and tone the muscles. Follow these with soothing effleurage to complete the treatment. End by moving your hands and yourself into position for the next phase of the massage.

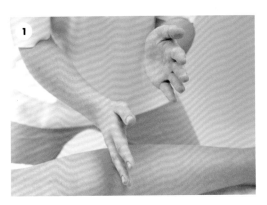

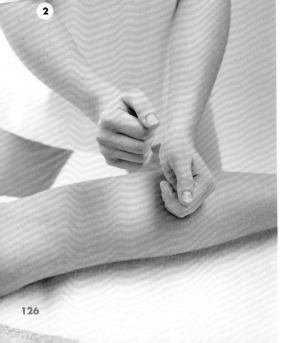

Hacking

1 *Apply firm and rhythmic hacking strokes with the outer edge of the hands all the way up the leg.*

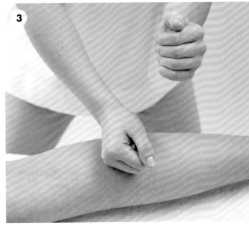

Pounding

2, 3 *Use closed fists alternately to apply pounding strokes up the back of the leg.*

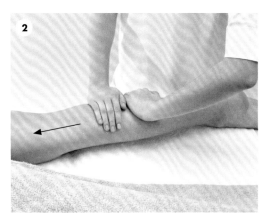

2

Effleurage
4 *Apply effleurage strokes to the whole leg from calf to thigh. Cover the leg and move to the other side to treat the other leg in the same way.*

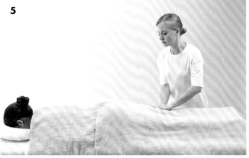

5

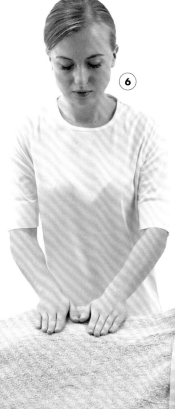

6

Cover & link
5, 6 *When you have treated both legs, cover the whole body and apply gliding effleurage linking strokes over the towels from the legs to the centre of the back.*

BACK The back comprises several complex structures that center on the bony column of the spine. The spine consists of 33 separate bones, known as vertebrae, which are connected by a system of joints to provide flexibility. Stability is provided by ligaments that support the joints in position. The ribcage is joined to the vertebrae in the upper part of the spine. Movement of the spine is generated by layers of muscles, symmetrically arranged on each side of the spine, from the deep muscles between the vertebrae to the mid layer and upper layer sheets of muscle. No muscles cross the spine. Although it is possible to perform a useful back massage without detailed knowledge of the anatomy, it is worth making a study of the detail of the structures in the back to gain a deeper understanding.

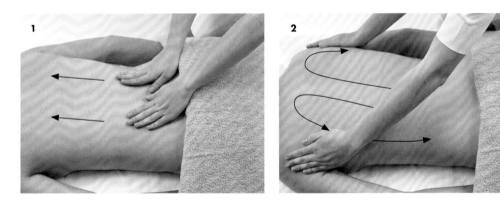

Effleurage

1, 2 *Place one hand on either side of the spine at the waist and apply a gliding effleurage stroke up the back, over the shoulders, and down the sides in a heart-shaped movement. Repeat three times.*

3

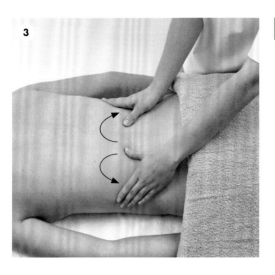

Massage of the Back

Massage of the back is one of the most appreciated sequences of a full-body massage, and is frequently done as a separate treatment. Back massage can provide relief from many types of backache, by releasing muscle tension and stiffness, which can compress nerves or inhibit mobility.

Never offer massage to anyone who has suffered a back injury until their doctor or medical specialist has confirmed that it is safe to do so.

Thumb pressure
3 *Place your thumbs about 1 inch (2.5 cm) on either side of the spine. Using the weight of your body to apply pressure, make circular movements with the thumbs. Repeat as you move your hands up the back to the neck.*

4

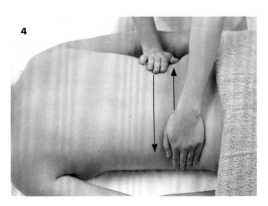

5

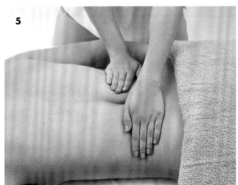

Wringing
4, 5 *Place your hands on either side of the back in the waist area. Using pressure, bring the hands toward each other and then back again. Repeat six times.*

Continued overleaf

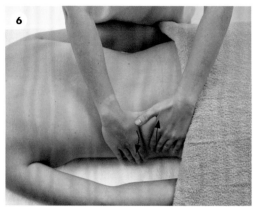

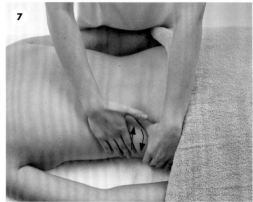

Kneading

6, 7, 8 *Working on one side, use both hands to knead the flesh of the waist area on the far side. Keep your hands moving in circles and move to the other side of the body and repeat the kneading on the other side.*

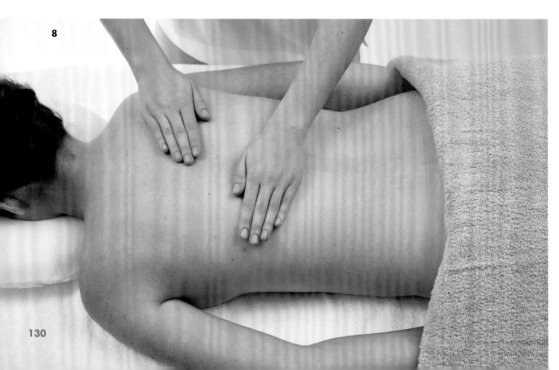

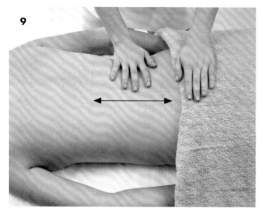

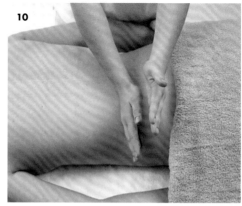

Vibration
9 *Apply firm pressure at the base of the spine with one hand, while using the other hand to make brisk vibrating movements up the back on one side and then down the back on the other side.*

Hacking
10 *Use hacking strokes on the fleshy sides of the lower back in the waist area. Work on both sides in turn.*

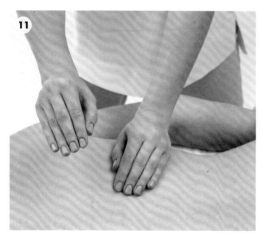

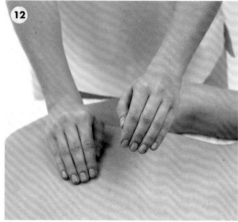

Cupping
11, 12 *Make a cup with both palms and tap from the lower back on one side and down the other side.*

SHOULDERS

The shoulder girdles are the paired structures that join the arms to the torso, marking the division between the back and the neck. Each shoulder girdle comprises a collarbone (clavicle) and a shoulder blade (scapula). The collarbones are joined to the top of the breast bone (sternum). The main muscles of the shoulder are the trapezius muscles. These triangular sheets of muscle join the shoulder joint to the spine from the middle of the back to the base of the skull. Deeper muscles control the movement of the shoulder blades.

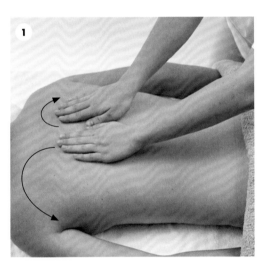

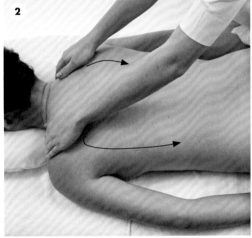

Effleurage

1, 2 *Apply three effleurage strokes in a continuous movement from the lower back to the shoulders, around the shoulders, and down the back again.*

Stress Relief

As well as being vulnerable to strain from excessive movement or exercise, the trapezius muscles can easily become a focus for mental stress. When we feel tense, it is a natural physical response to hunch our shoulders and over time this can lead to pain and stiffness. Massage can be a huge benefit in such cases.

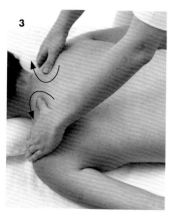

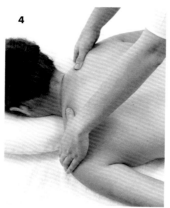

Thumb pressure
3, 4 *Use the thumbs on both hands to apply pressure in small circular movements over both shoulders.*

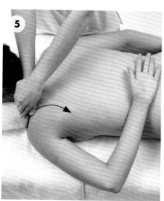

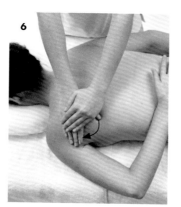

Scapula lift
5, 6 *Cross the arm farthest from you over the back, palm up. Apply pressure with one hand over the other to the top of the shoulder blade of the bent arm. Move your hands to treat the whole shoulder blade area. Change to the other side and repeat.*

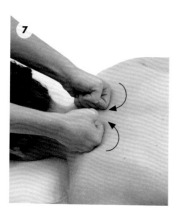

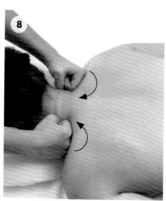

Fist pressure
7, 8 *Apply circular pressure with the fists on both shoulders, moving from the upper back to the tops of the shoulders.*

BACK OF NECK & SCALP

The neck is formed of the upper seven vertebrae of the spinal column, termed the cervical vertebrae. These bones are usually easily felt during massage. The trapezius muscles join each side of the back of the neck. Massage of this area is an extension of treatment of the shoulder, but it also specifically addresses the strains that may arise from awkward or repetitive movements and poor posture. The neck contains vital blood vessels, so be sure to avoid excessive or prolonged pressure on any area. The final area to be treated in the face down position is the scalp. The flesh covering the skull is very thin, but contains many blood vessels and nerve endings. Massage of this area utilizes a variety of specialized strokes, which are both stimulating and relaxing for the receiver. Take care not to pull the hair sharply while you are working, as this could negate the benefits.

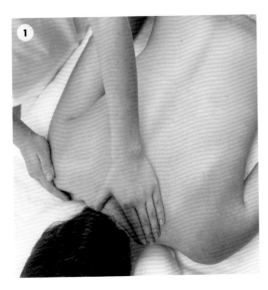

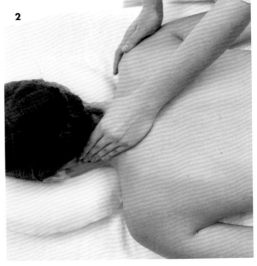

Caterpillar

1 Use one hand to squeeze the flesh at the back of the neck, pulling it up and away from the bone. Do this three times.

Thumb pressure

2 Squeezing the base of the head with your thumb and fingers, make small circular movements on either side. End with a connecting effleurage stroke of the whole back.

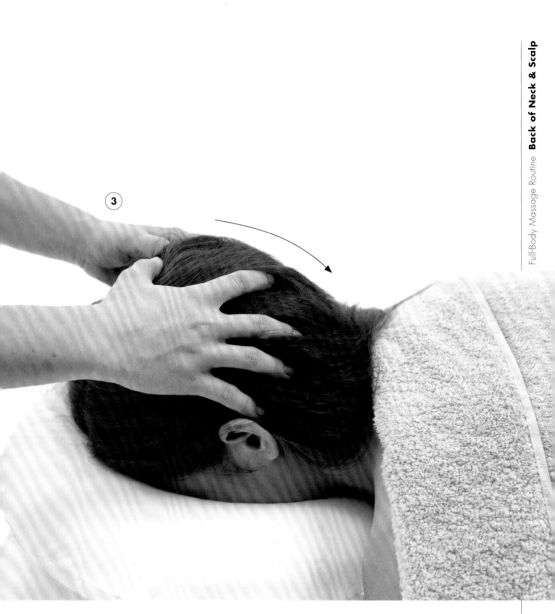

Combing

3 *Place your hands on the head and make alternate combing movements through the hair from the front to the back of the head. Emphasize working through the hair and concentrate on the scalp, using the pads of the fingers.*

Continued overleaf

135

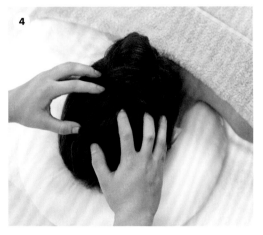

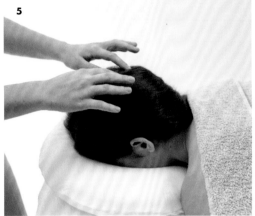

Shampooing
4 *Using both hands, make shampooing movements through the hair.*

Scalp flicks
5 *Using the fingers of both hands, pluck the scalp all over.*

Raindrops
6 *Lightly tap the fingers of both hands all over the scalp, working on the scalp with the pads of the fingertips.*

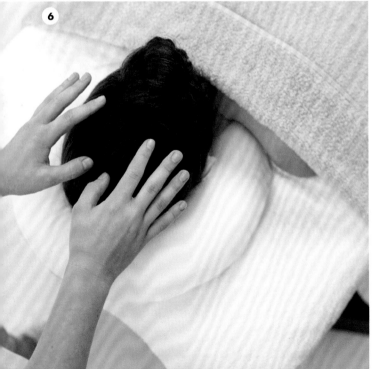

Hair grabs
7 *Gently but firmly use both hands to pull handfuls of hair all over the scalp.*

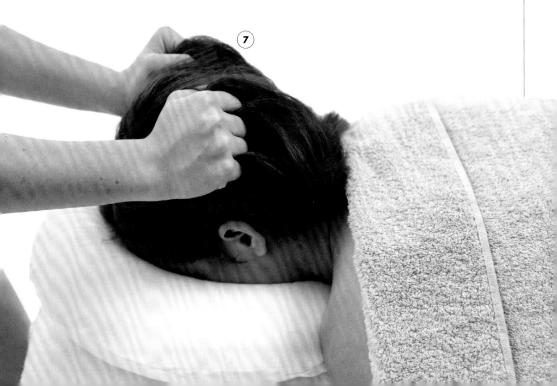

Phase 2 • Face Up

For the second phase of the massage, the receiver moves to a face-up position on the massage table. Help the person remain modestly covered as they turn around by holding a large towel just over them while they change position. Be sure to avert your gaze as you do so.

Once the person is comfortably settled in the face-up position, rearrange the towels—one draped over the upper part of the body and the other over the lower half. Once more, check that they are lying as symmetrically as possible, and carefully adjust their position if necessary.

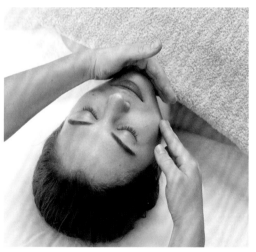 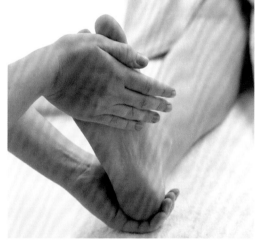

From head to toe
The face-up phase starts with the face and moves down the body to end with a foot massage.

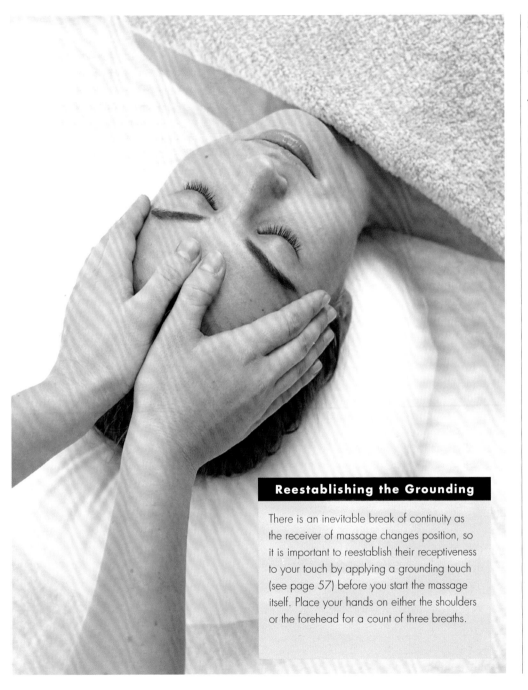

Reestablishing the Grounding

There is an inevitable break of continuity as the receiver of massage changes position, so it is important to reestablish their receptiveness to your touch by applying a grounding touch (see page 57) before you start the massage itself. Place your hands on either the shoulders or the forehead for a count of three breaths.

FACE The nerves that serve the face and the facial muscles are very receptive to massage. There is no significant muscle bulk that you can treat with the more vigorous massage strokes, but the application of pressure at various points is highly effective. Headaches and sinus congestion are among the conditions that may be improved by facial massage. The circulation-stimulating effect of massage has significant benefits for the condition and appearance of the skin of the face.

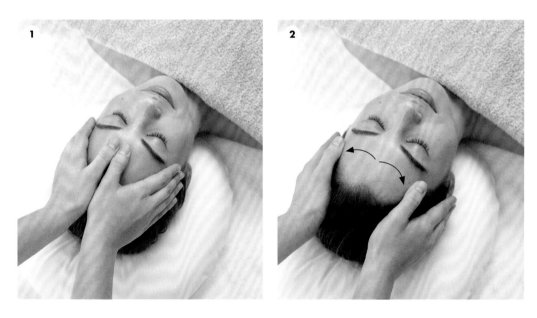

Smoothing
1, 2 *Place the thumbs of both hands close together in the center of the forehead and hold for a count of three. Then move the thumbs apart in a smoothing movement to each side of the forehead.*

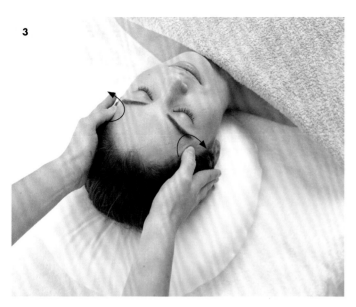

Thumb pressure—temples

3 *Apply pressure with the thumbs in small circling movements around the temples.*

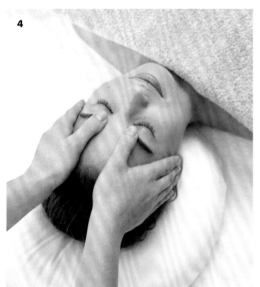

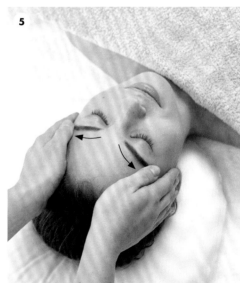

Thumb pressure—eyebrows

4, 5 *Apply thumb pressure from the inner to the outer edge of the eyebrows.*

Continued overleaf

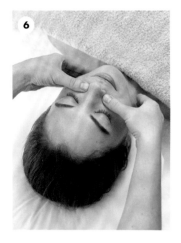 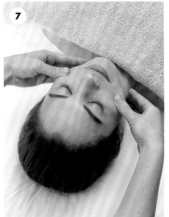 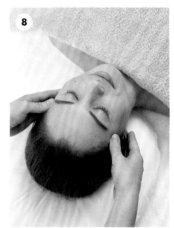

Nose & cheeks

6, 7, 8 *Apply circling thumb pressure on either side of the nose, moving the thumbs outward to pull up under the cheekbone, finishing at the temples. Repeat three times.*

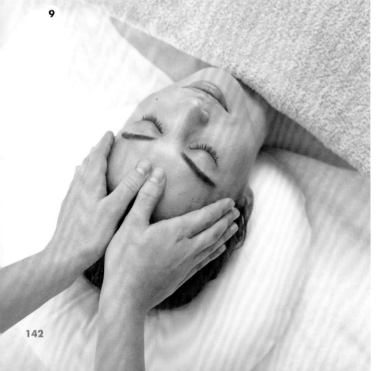

Third-eye position

9 *Move your thumbs to the center of the forehead, known as the third-eye position. Keep your hands flat on the sides of the forehead and apply gradually increasing pressure with your thumbs.*

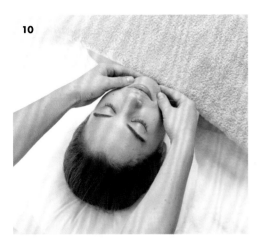

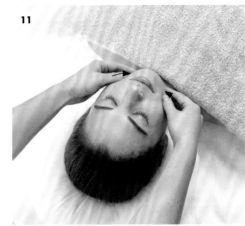

Massaging the jawbone

10, 11 *Use your fingers to press along the underside of the jawbone from sides to center.*

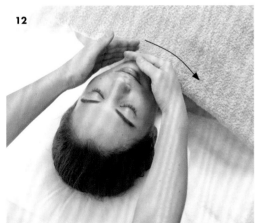

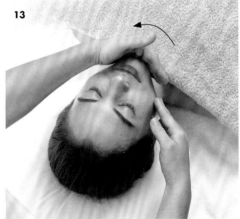

Effleurage

12, 13 *Apply effleurage strokes with your fingers together under and around the chin from the center to the outer edge alternately in each direction. Repeat three times. End with your thumbs in the third-eye position (step 9).*

NECK & UPPER CHEST
This phase of the massage sequence starts with the upper chest, the bony area between the collarbones and the breast area. Although not significantly muscled, emotional stress can create tension in this area and gentle strokes can allow opening of the chest and more effective breathing. The sequence then revisits the back of the neck (the throat is not massaged). The change in angle of working allows for gentle stretching and freeing of the joints between the cervical vertebrae and the muscles that surround the neck and help to support the head.

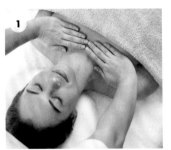

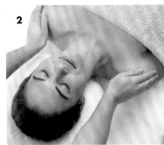

Upper chest

1, 2, 3, 4 *Place both hands, fingertips together, on the upper chest. Apply moderate pressure. Move your hands outward and around to the shoulder in a flowing movement. End by cupping the shoulders. Then glide the backs of the hands over the shoulder. Repeat three times.*

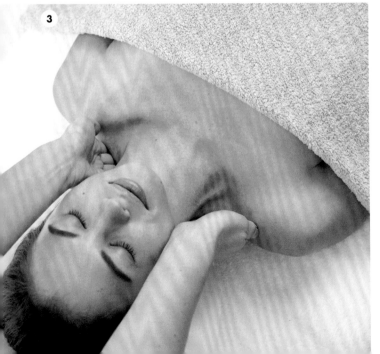

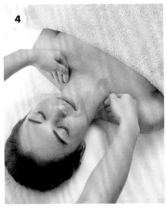

Finger pressure

5, 6, *Apply pressure with the index finger of each hand alternately under the neck on either side of the spine. Work upward from the base of the neck to the base of the skull.*

5

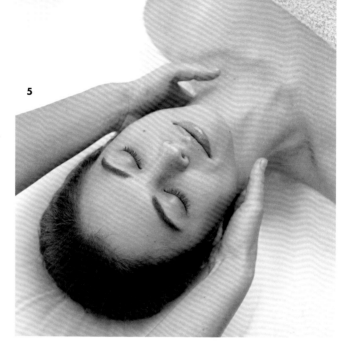

6

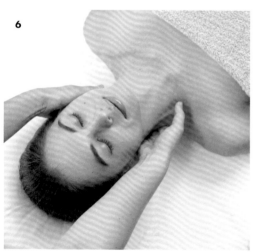

7

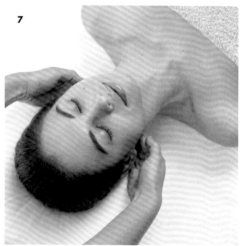

Circling pressure

7 *Using your fingertips, apply circling pressure to the muscles at the base of the skull.*

Continued overleaf

145

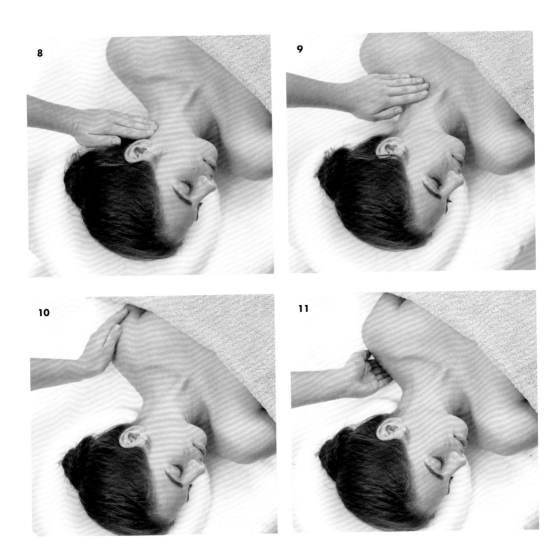

Sides of neck

8, 9, 10, 11 *Turn the head to one side. Place the fingertips of one hand on the side of the neck below the ear. Using gentle pressure, move the fingertips down the neck and along and behind the shoulder. Repeat three times. Turn the head to the other side and repeat steps 8 to 11.*

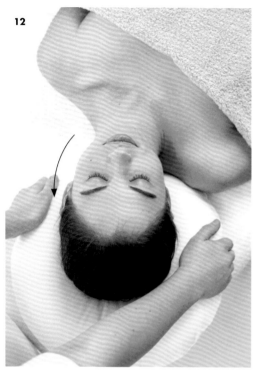

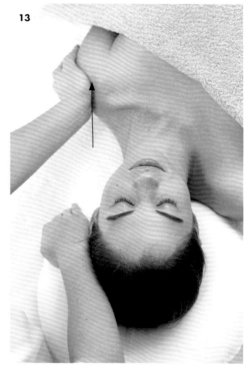

Neck stretch

12, 13 *Move the head support to one side. Push down the shoulder with one hand, keeping the head to one side with the other hand and arm. Hold for three seconds and relax three times. Repeat steps 12 to 13 on the other side.*

HAND

The hands and wrists are among the most hard-working parts of the body. They are in almost constant use—holding, manipulating, and supporting. The numerous tiny bones and joints of the hands and fingers are vulnerable to problems related to overuse, such as repetitive strain injury, and degenerative conditions, such as the various forms of arthritis. Massage can help ease the pain and disability associated with these conditions by mobilizing the joints and boosting circulation.

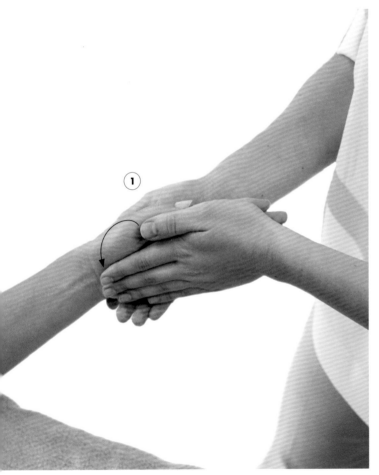

Effleurage of the palm
1 *After grounding for a few moments through the towel, support the side of the receiver's hand with one hand. Place your other hand against the palm and make circular movements.*

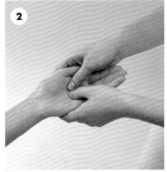

Thumb pressure
2 *Apply pressure with the thumbs, using circular movements, around the whole palm area.*

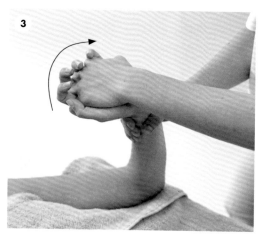

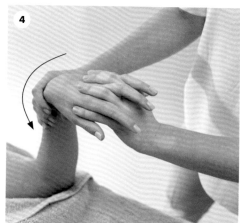

Wrist rotations

3, 4 *Hold the arm just below the wrist with one hand. Interlace the fingers of your other hand with the receiver's. Rotate the wrist clockwise and then counterclockwise.*

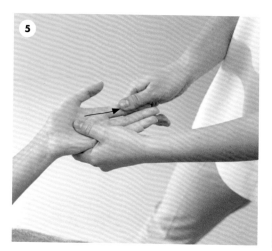

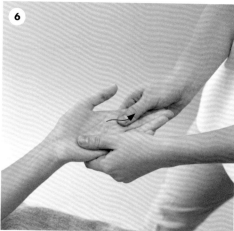

Finger pulls

5, 6 *With the palm upward, gently pull each finger and thumb while steadying the receiver's hand with your other hand. Repeat steps 1 to 6 on the receiver's other hand.*

FOREARM

The forearm, the part of the arm from the elbow to the wrist, consists of a pair of bones, the radius and the ulna, which are enclosed within several distinct muscles attached to the elbow and wrists. These muscles control the movement of the wrist and, like any other skeletal muscles, can become stiff, swollen, and painful when overused. Swelling of these muscles can compress the median nerve that passes through this area, leading to further pain and reduced wrist function. Light- and medium-pressure strokes help to counteract many problems.

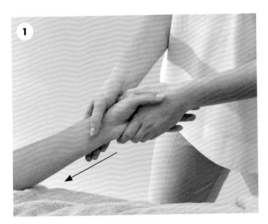

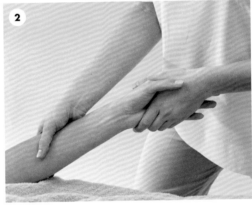

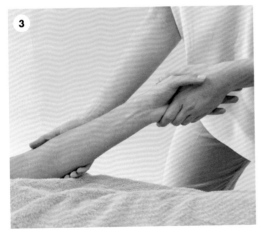

Effleurage

1, 2, 3 Support the receiver's hand with one hand. Use your other hand to give effleurage strokes from wrist to elbow.

4

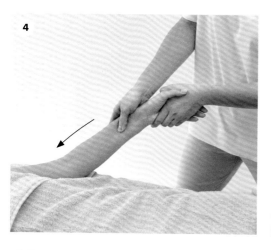

5

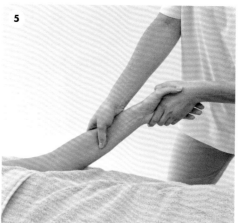

Sliding squeeze
4, 5 *Squeeze the forearm between the thumb and fingers in a one-handed caterpillar squeeze, while sliding the hand down from wrist to elbow.*

Circling thumb pressure
6 *Apply thumb pressure in a circulating movement down the inside of the forearm from wrist to elbow. Move on to the upper arm (overleaf) before switching to the other arm.*

6

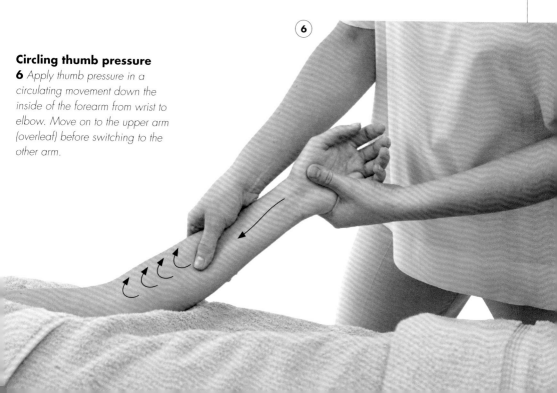

UPPER ARM

The core of the upper arm, which extends from the shoulder joint to the elbow, is the humerus bone. The powerful biceps muscle at the front of the arm controls bending of the elbow and lifting of the forearm. The triceps muscle at the back of the arm is responsible for straightening the arm. Additional smaller muscles create twisting movements of the arm. Almost all of us use our arms constantly for lifting and carrying, whether at home, at work, or while engaged in sport. Stiff and aching upper arm muscles respond well to a variety of massage strokes.

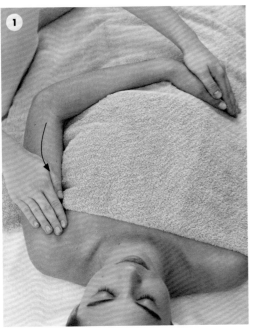 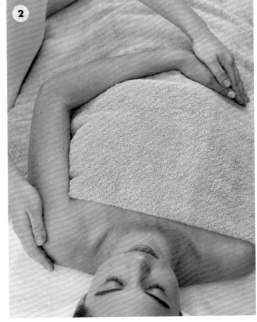

Effleurage
1, 2 *With the elbow bent and the forearm placed across the body, give effleurage strokes from elbow to shoulder. Repeat three times.*

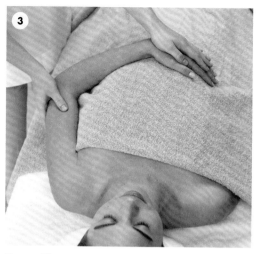

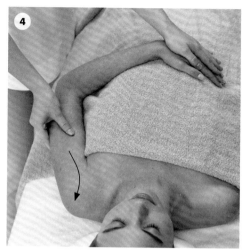

Caterpillar squeeze
3, 4 *Apply caterpillar squeezes from elbow to shoulder. Repeat three times.*

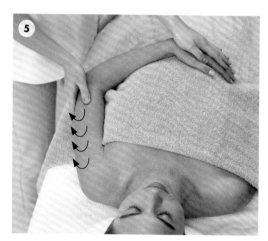

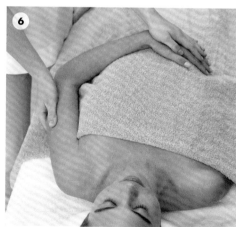

Thumb pressure
5, 6 *Apply thumb pressure in small circular movements along the upper surface of the arm. Move the arm farther across the body to allow you to treat the underside of the arm in the same way. Repeat the forearm and upper arm massages on the other arm.*

Belly

The belly, or abdomen, contains most of the digestive organs. The area is covered by sheets of muscle—commonly known as "abs." Other muscles in this part of the body include the muscles between the ribs—the intercostal muscles. The aim of massage in this area is not only to relax and tone these skeletal muscles, but also to gently stimulate the digestive organs beneath. The direction of the strokes—clockwise—is important as it harmonizes with the direction of the waves of muscular contractions of the digestive tract from the stomach through the intestines.

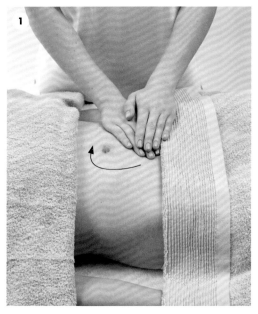

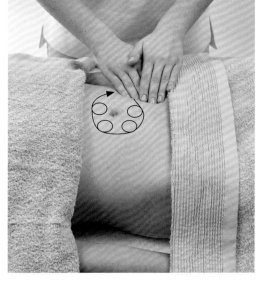

Effleurage

1 *Fold back the towel to expose the area between the ribs and the pelvis and with one hand over the other, make effleurage movements in a clockwise direction around the belly area.*

Circling pressure

2 *Make small circling movements in a clockwise direction over the whole area. Be careful to adjust the pressure for the comfort of the receiver.*

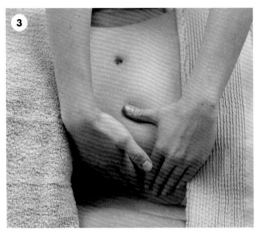

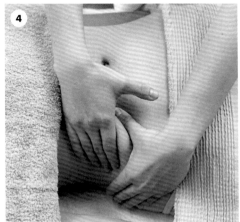

Kneading

3, 4 *Knead the side of the belly area farthest from you. Keeping both hands in contact with the receiver, move around to the other side and repeat the kneading on that side.*

Intercostal massage

5 *Place your hands over the ribs on both sides. Locate the fingers between the ribs and drag the hands upward over the intercostal muscles. Replace the towel over the belly.*

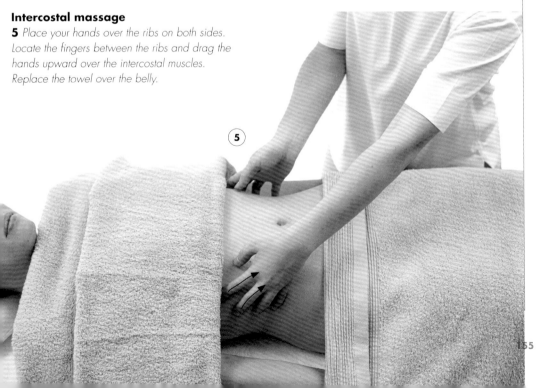

FRONT OF THIGH

The key feature of the front of the thigh is the powerful muscle group known as the quadriceps (popularly called the "quads"). These are joined to the knee and the pelvis. Contraction of these muscles extends the leg. They work particularly hard when we climb stairs, for example, or undertake similar actions in which the leg is straightened while supporting the weight of the body. Massage helps to relax and tone these muscles, and is especially useful both before and after sporting activities.

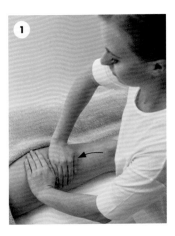

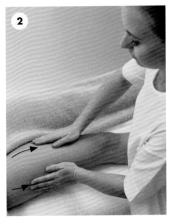

Effleurage

1, 2 *Fold back the towel on one side. Using both hands, apply circulating effleurage strokes upward from the knee to the top of the thigh and, separating the hands, down each side along the sides of the thigh.*

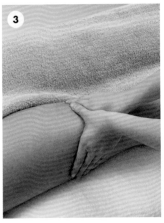

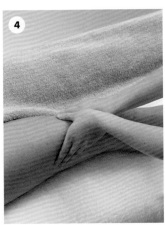

Caterpillar squeeze

3, 4 *Use both hands to alternately pluck and pull the flesh, working from above the knee toward the upper thigh. Repeat three times.*

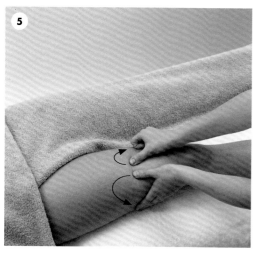

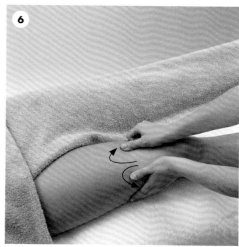

Thumb pressure

5, 6 *Apply circling thumb pressure from above the knee to the upper thigh.*

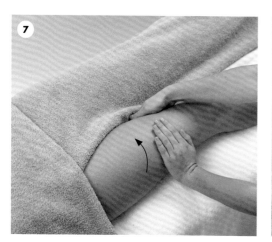

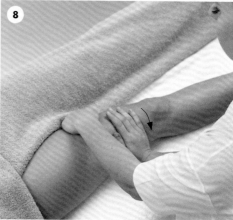

Wringing

7, 8 *Use the hands working in opposite directions to apply a wringing action across the thigh. Treat the whole thigh upward from the knee. Move on to the knee and front of the lower leg (overleaf) before switching to the other leg.*

KNEE & FRONT OF LOWER LEG

The knee is essentially a hinge joint between the femur (thigh bone) and the main bone of the lower leg, the tibia (shin bone). The joint is protected at the front by a "floating" bone, the patella (kneecap). It is surrounded by a complex network of tendons and ligaments that anchor the muscles of the thigh and lower leg. Below the knee, the tibia is joined on its outer side to a smaller bone, the fibula. This pair of bones extend to the ankle. The muscles of the front of the lower leg are relatively thin, but along with the tendons that surround the knee, are softened and eased by massage.

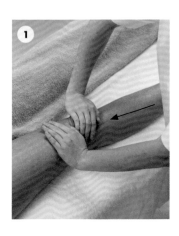

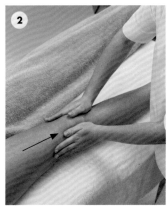

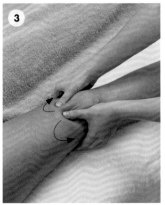

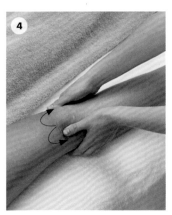

Knee effleurage

1, 2 *Apply circling effleurage strokes from just below to just above the knee and down along the sides of the knee.*

Thumb pressure

3, 4 *Apply circling thumb pressure around the kneecap, starting at the center and working outward. Repeat effleurage as in steps 1 and 2.*

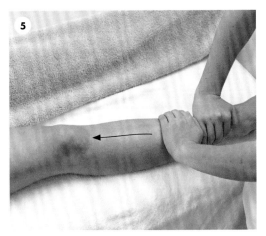

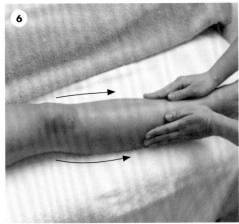

Effleurage of the lower leg

5, 6 *Apply two-handed circling effleurage strokes over the front of the lower leg from ankle to knee, and bring the hands back down each side of the calf.*

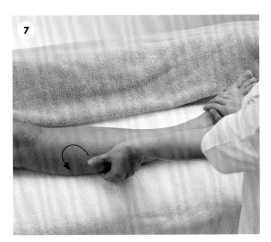

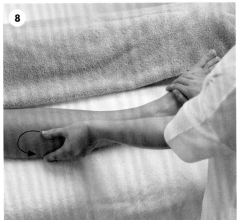

Thumb pressure

7, 8 *Support the foot with one hand and use the thumb of the other hand to apply circling pressure over the outer side of the lower leg from ankle to knee. Keep the pressure light. Repeat the front of thigh, knee and lower leg massages on the other leg.*

ANKLES & FEET

The ankle joint is formed at the meeting point of the two bones of the lower leg, the tibia and fibula, and the multiple bones of the upper part of the foot and heel, known as the tarsals. The tarsals are rigidly joined to the five metatarsals, which are, in effect, the origin of the toes. The joint between each toe and its metatarsal is flexible, as are the individual joints of the toes. This complex arrangement of small bones and joints is highly receptive to the benefits of massage, which can help to relieve pain and discomfort caused by long periods of standing, walking, or running, and from the pressures of inappropriate or ill-fitting footwear.

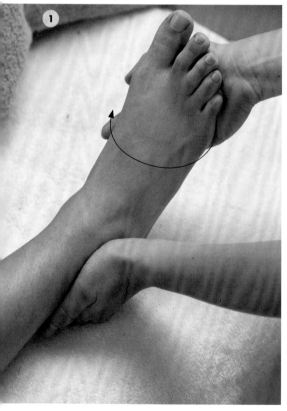

Ankle rotations

1, 2 *Hold the foot in one hand and support the heel with the other hand. Rotate the ankle in each direction.*

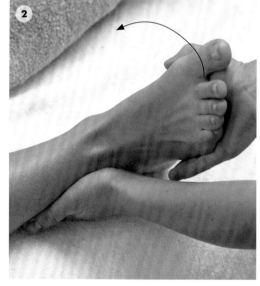

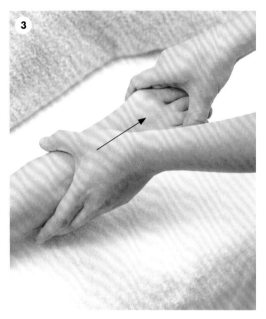

Effleurage
3, 4, 5 *Gently apply effleurage strokes to the front of the foot from ankle to toes, using each hand alternately.*

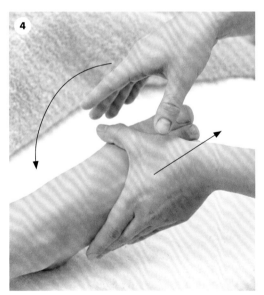

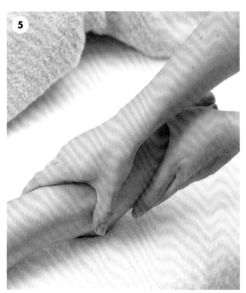

Continued overleaf

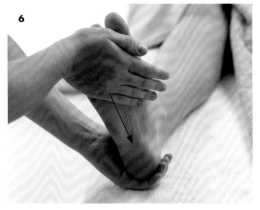

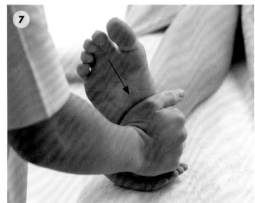

Heel-of-hand pressure

6, 7 *Support the foot in one hand and use the heel of the other hand to apply medium-pressure strokes to the sole of the foot from toes to heel.*

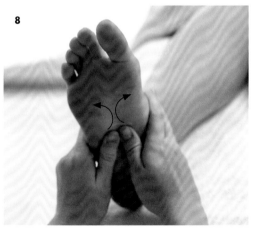

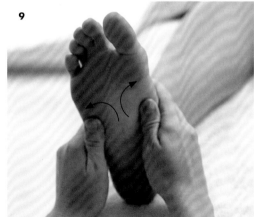

Thumb pressure

8, 9 *Apply thumb pressure to the sole of the foot, working outward from the middle in small, circular movements.*

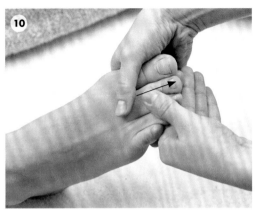

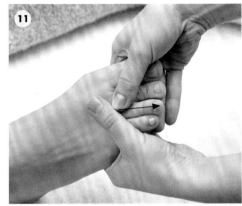

Toe tugs

10, 11 *Alternating hands and with rhythmical movement, pull each toe from its base using one hand while using the other hand to provide support.*

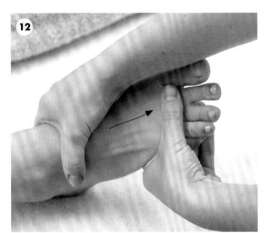

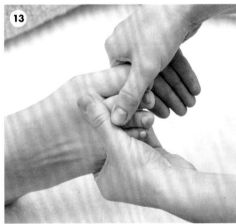

Foot pulls

12, 13 *Alternating hands and with rhythmical movement, pull from the top of the ankle towards the toes. Repeat three times and then repeat steps 1 to 13 on the other foot.*

163

SPECIFIC MASSAGES

You can use your massage skills to address specific issues or needs, as well as to provide a generalized health-enhancing therapy. In this chapter, you will be introduced to focused treatment routines that can be used to alleviate problems in a particular area of the body or in particular circumstances, such as after sport. The final section teaches techniques for self-massage, which can be useful for instant relief of stresses and strains when you are without access to a massage partner.

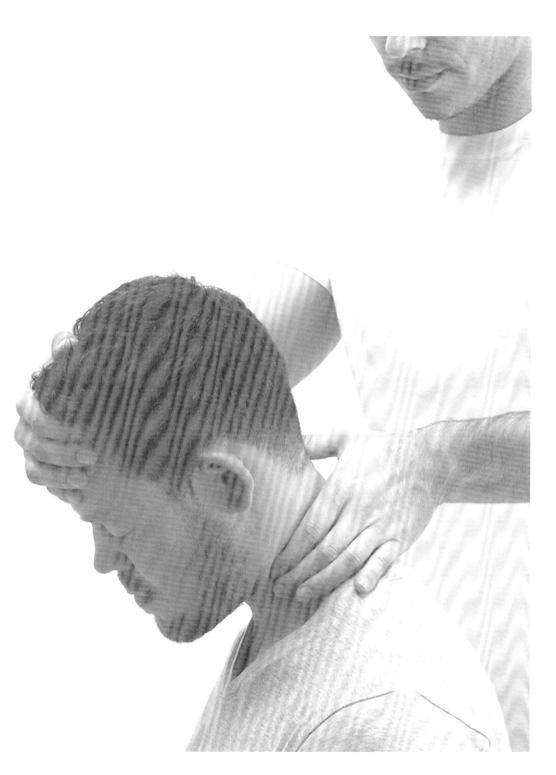

SCALP & FACE

The head, with its rich supply of nerve endings and blood vessels, can be a focus for stress-related tension. Many of us today spend long hours staring at computer screens or at printouts, leading to what is commonly termed eyestrain, but is more accurately the consequence of overworking the muscles around the eyes and in the head area in general. Tension headaches are often the result.

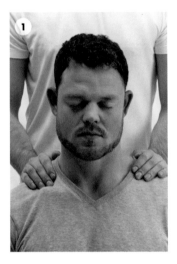

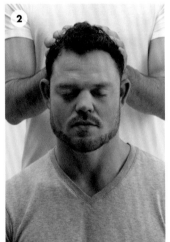

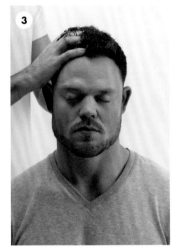

Grounding

1 *With the receiver sitting upright in a chair, rest your hands on the shoulders and focus for a few moments.*

Combing

2, 3 *Run your fingers through the hair and across the scalp as if combing the hair.*

Indian Head Massage

Traditional Indian approaches to health maintenance include head massage as a valued part of a regular health and beauty routine. Stimulation of the blood supply in the scalp is thought to contribute to healthy activity of the hair follicles. Western classical massage therapists have learned from this tradition and often incorporate this practice into their routines. Head massage can be an ideal "quick fix" when a full massage is not feasible. For a traditional Indian head massage, you would use oils scented with essential oils such as jasmine or neroli. But this is a matter of personal choice.

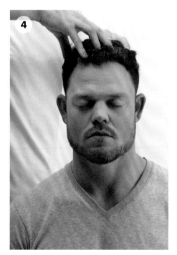

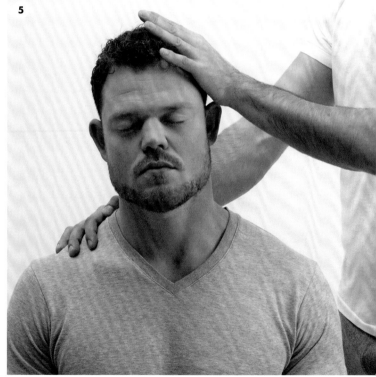

Shampooing
4 *Use both hands to rub the scalp as if shampooing the hair.*

Ruffling
5 *Vigorously ruffle the hair all over with the palm of your hand, applying firm pressure to the scalp.*

Continued overleaf

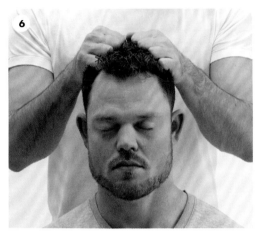

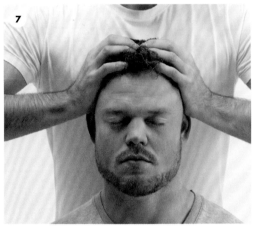

Hair grabs
6 Grab handfuls of hair and circle with the heels of the hand against the scalp. Work over the entire scalp.

Side-to-side squeeze
7 With the palms of your hands, apply pressure to the sides of the head for a count of three.

Front-to-back squeeze
8 With the palms of your hands, apply pressure to the forehead and back of the head for a count of three.

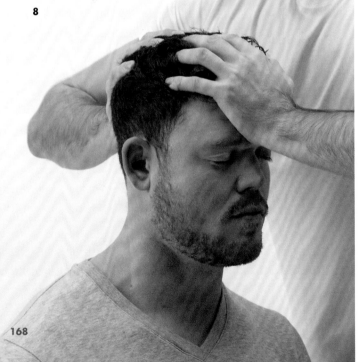

9

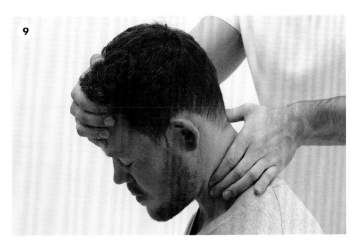

Base of skull pressure

9 *Support the forehead with one hand and place the thumb in the indentation at the base of the skull. Apply pressure for a count of three.*

Third-eye pressure

10 *Hold the third-eye position as you count to three gradually release the pressure*

10

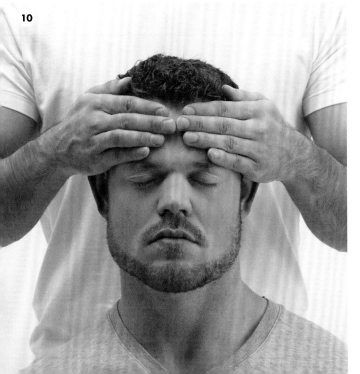

Continued overleaf

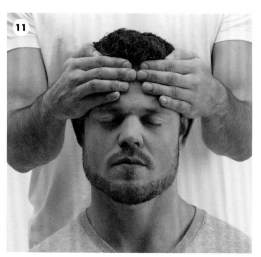

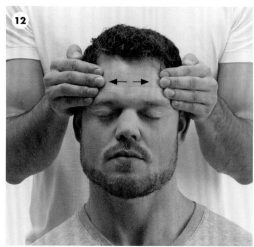

Smoothing the forehead

11, 12 *Place both hands on the forehead, fingertips together, and press the center of the forehead for a count of three with gradually increasing pressure. Pull the hands apart in a smoothing action.*

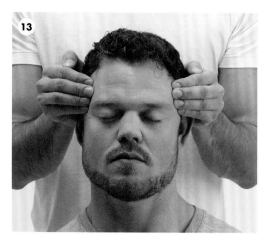

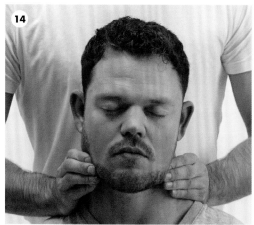

Temple circling

13 *Apply circling pressure to the temples with your fingertips for a count of three.*

Jaw circling

14 *Place the fingertips on the jaw under the cheekbones and apply circing pressure with your fingertips.*

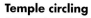

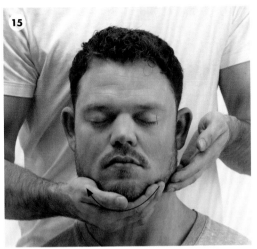

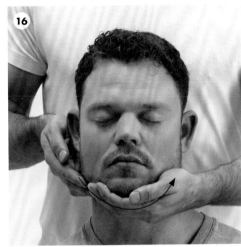

Jaw effleurage

15, 16 *Slide down toward the chin. Cup the chin in one hand and slide both hands around in alternating movements. Finish by repeating the third-eye pressure (10 and 11). Repeat three times.*

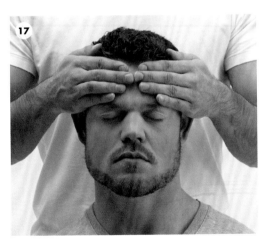

Third-eye pressure

17 *Finish with the third-eye position, holding while you count to three and gradually release the pressure*

SHOULDERS & NECK

Sitting in a hunched position, particularly when wrestling with a difficult work problem at a desk, is a typical cause of tightness in the muscles of the neck and shoulders. The muscles become tense and inflexible, the shoulders rise up toward the ears, and the whole area can feel stiff and painful. A massage that focuses on this area is one of the most sought-after and useful specific massages. By concentrating on loosening knots and stretching the muscles in this area, a massage therapist can help to alleviate the severe posture problems that can arise out of a long-term neglect of this form of tension. For this classic workplace massage, the receiver of the massage is seated and clothed. Always start with a few moments of grounding by placing your hands on the receiver's shoulders.

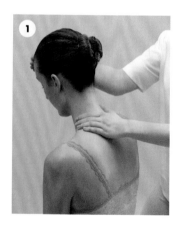 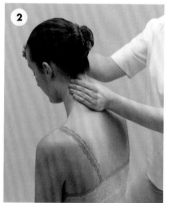 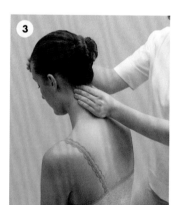

Caterpillar squeezes
1 *Support the forehead with one hand, and use the other to apply caterpillar squeezes up the back of the neck.*

Thumb pressure
2, 3 *Apply circling pressure with your thumbs on each side of the spine at the base of the skull.*

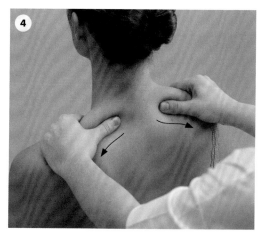

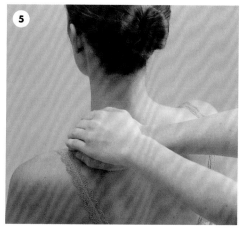

Trapezius squeezes
4 *Squeeze the trapezius between the thumb and fingers, working outward from the neck.*

Trapezius pulls
5 *With one hand on top of the other, pull the trapezius back and repeat on the other shoulder.*

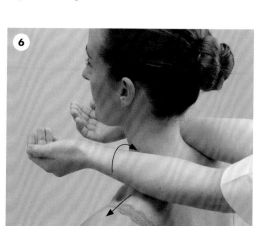

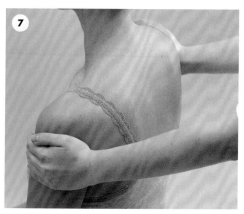

Shoulder presses
6 *Press down on both shoulders with the back of the forearms, bending your knees to use your body weight to apply pressure. As you do so, roll your forearms in and move them outward toward the outer edge of the shoulders.*

Upper-arm squeeze
7 *Squeeze the upper arms with both hands for a count of three.*

Continued overleaf

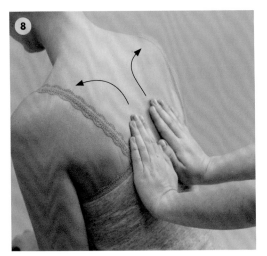

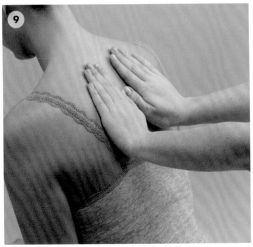

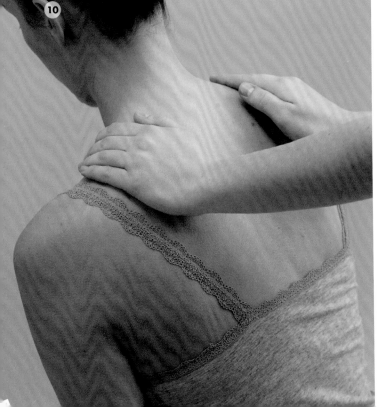

Back effleurage
8, 9, 10 *With the receiver leaning forward, apply effleurage strokes up the length of the back.*

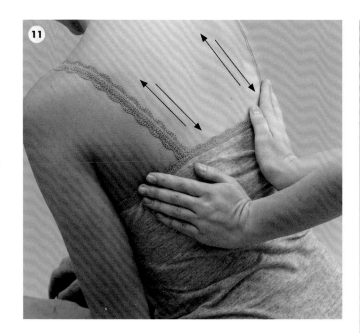

Palm pressure

11 *Using both hands, apply alternating palm pressure down the back on either side of the spine. Work back up the spine and follow with effleurage strokes down the back.*

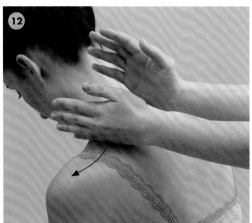

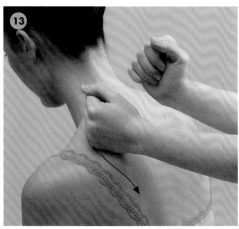

Shoulder hacking

12 *Apply hacking strokes with the outer edges of both hands along the trapezius muscle at the top of each shoulder.*

Shoulder pounding

13 *Use your closed fists to apply pounding strokes down the upper back, working down and then up on each side, then finish with effleurage.*

WRISTS & HANDS

Even those who lead a sedentary life are constantly moving their hands and wrists, parts of the body that incorporate some of our most complex networks of bones and joints. In some circumstances, this workload alone can lead to strain and discomfort. Problems in this area can be exacerbated by fluid retention resulting from hormonal changes, which can cause painful constriction of the nerve pathways, and by joint changes caused by osteoarthritis. Massage, including gentle stretching to ease the joints, can provide relief, if not a cure, for many of these conditions. And gentle manipulation of the hands is often soothing and comforting to those who cannot tolerate a full massage.

Dry Hands

Grounding
1 *Hold the receiver's hand, palm upward, between both your palms for a count of three.*

Because the hands are often dry, it is a good idea to use oil for this massage. Treat both hands in the same way.

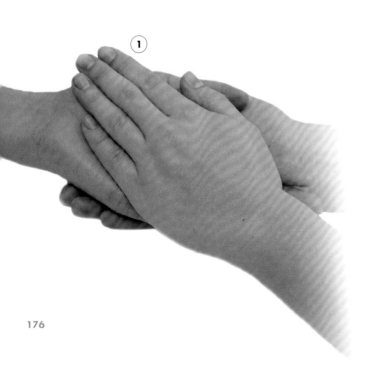

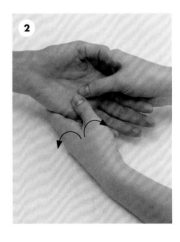

Thumb pressure
2 *Apply circling pressure with the thumbs to all areas of the palm.*

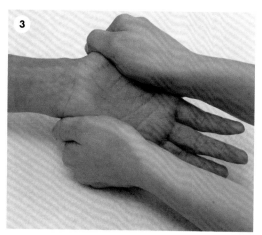

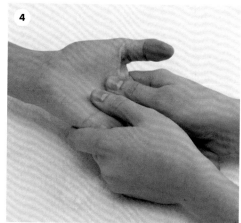

Palm stretch
3 *Hold each side of the receiver's hand and use both hands to gently bend the palm outward.*

Palm wriggling
4 *Keeping your thumbs parallel, apply pressure in an up and down movement from one side of the palm to the other.*

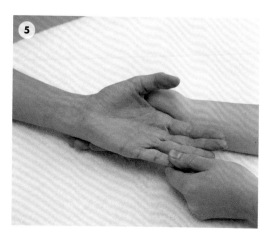

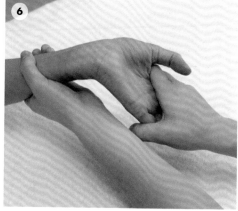

Finger pulls
5 *Pull each of the fingers in turn, firmly but gently. Do not aim to make the joints "click."*

Forearm stretch
6 *Supporting the forearm with one hand, bend the receiver's hand backward as far as is comfortable. Repeat steps 1 to 6 for the receiver's other hand.*

FEET It goes without saying that massage of the feet after a long walk or a long period of standing will provide welcome relief of aches and pains. But many complementary therapists believe that massage of specific areas of the foot can do much more, providing health benefits in other areas of the body. This approach is known as reflexology. The details of reflexology theory are beyond the scope of this book, and practitioners of classic massage do not necessarily have to adhere to all the theories underlying this system to incorporate some of its teaching into their practice. What is beyond doubt is that a careful and thorough foot massage can leave a person feeling both relaxed and energized.

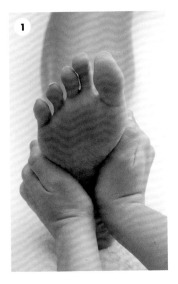
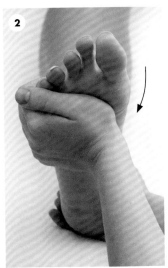
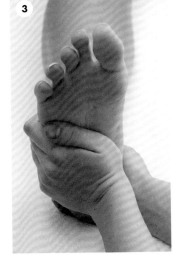

Grounding
1 *Start with grounding by enclosing the foot in both hands for a count of three.*

Effleurage
2, 3 *Apply effleurage strokes from toe to heel with the heel of the hand.*

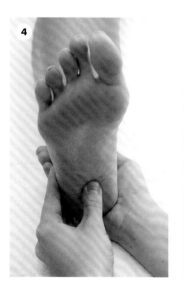 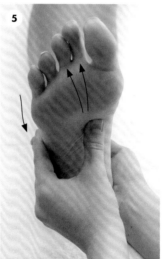 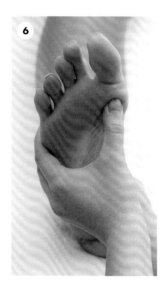

Thumb pressure

4, 5, 6 *Slide the thumb, using firm pressure, up the sole of the foot in a line from the heel to the base of the big toe. Repeat, following a line toward the base of each toe.*

Continued overleaf

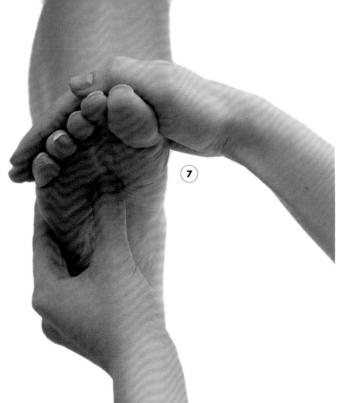

Central pressure

7 *Pull the foot toward you while applying thumb pressure in the indentation just below the center of the ball of the foot—the solar plexus point, according to reflexology.*

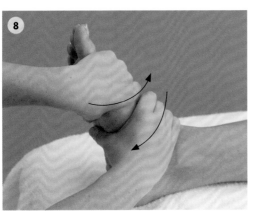

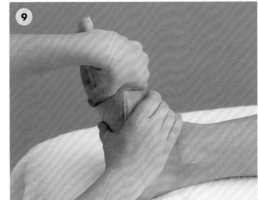

Foot twists

8, 9 *Grasping the foot with both hands, twist the hands in opposite directions to twist the foot in a wringing action. Repeat three times in each direction.*

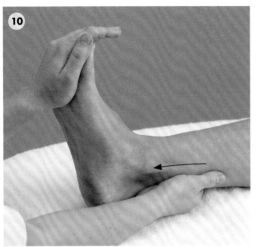

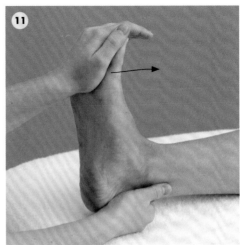

Calf stretch
10, 11, 12 *Hold the lower calf and slide your hand down toward the heel while pushing the foot and then the toes backward with the other hand. Repeat steps 1 to 12 on the other foot.*

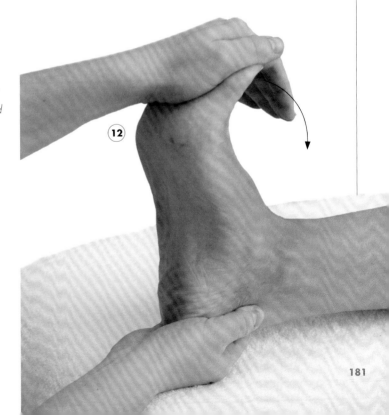

181

SPORTS MASSAGE

Over the years, massage has become established as an essential element in training and health maintenance programs for athletes and those engaged in sports of all kinds. There is wide recognition among specialist sports physiotherapists of the benefits that massage can provide, both in reducing the chances of injury and strain and in promoting recovery. Athletes and top sports teams include in their staff massage therapists who have been specially trained in specific techniques that address the types of problems likely to be experienced by elite sportsmen and women. But sports massage is not only appropriate for those performing at a high level. Anyone who engages in strenuous physical activity can benefit from thoughtfully applied massage strokes, both before and after an event or training session.

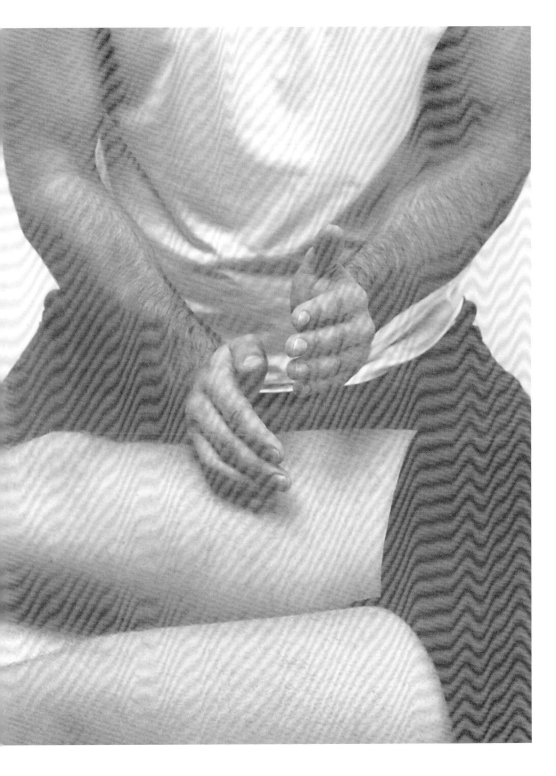

Pre- & Post-Event Massage

Although many of the techniques of sports massage are too specialized for a book of this kind, there are many that can be employed by a novice massage therapist to the advantage of the person they are treating. On the following pages, massage sequences designed to prepare the body for exertion—pre-event massage—and to maximize recovery afterward—post-event massage—are described.

Pre-event massage

Massage can be both stimulating and relaxing and these dual benefits come to the fore when preparing the body for a sporting event. In this situation, assuming there is no preexisting condition to be addressed (in such a case it may be advisable to counsel against participation), the primary aim will be to "wake up" the muscles and mind in readiness for exertion. A massage routine that emphasizes circulation-stimulating strokes, namely the various percussion strokes, is most appropriate. But the muscles and the surrounding connective tissues also need to be softened and relaxed in order to maximize their

elasticity and reduce the likelihood of strain and injury. This requires the inclusion of the soothing long strokes of effleurage and the muscle-stretching effect of light petrissage.

Post-event massage

After a strenuous sporting event, the muscles are likely to be both slightly swollen and stiff. The increased blood flow during physical activity can lead to swelling in muscle tissue, especially when small tears have occurred. Following exercise, such swelling may restrict the circulation of blood, leading to further swelling. Muscles can also become tense after a period of intense exercise, a natural response that is intended to protect them from further use.

Relaxing massage strokes can improve the circulation of blood through the muscles and, by stimulating the nerves, ease tension and stiffness, restoring muscle length and pliability.

Addressing Knots

When a muscle or group of muscles have been strained or perhaps damaged, resulting in small tears in the muscle fibers, the result can be areas of "knottiness" — where the muscles have gone into spasm to protect the area. In some cases, such knots may be caused by the formation of tiny areas of inflexible scar tissue within a previously damaged muscle. When performing a massage, you may come across these areas of stiffness, where the muscles do not readily soften in response to your touch. The person you are treating may also notice discomfort as you work that area. Such muscle knots may benefit from specific massage strokes. But do not continue to massage that area if it causes more than slight discomfort that increases rather than easing following your touch.

PRE-EVENT MASSAGE

Much of the general massage sequence described in the previous chapter can be used for pre-event massage, but the pace and rhythm should be more brisk. Here, the focus is on sequences that have specific benefits before a sporting event. The overall rhythm of the massage is brisk. And, if the receiver agrees, you can choose to use lubricating oil scented with essential oils that have an invigorating effect, such as ginger or sandalwood.

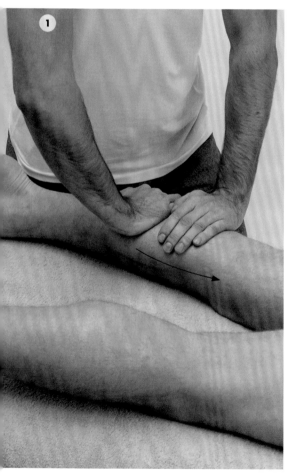

Two-handed effleurage

1, 2 *Using both hands together, apply sliding strokes from ankle to thigh, and gently slide back toward the ankle. Repeat five times.*

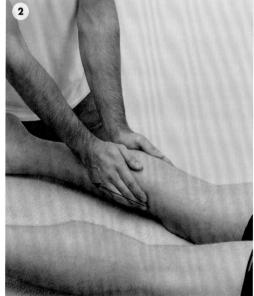

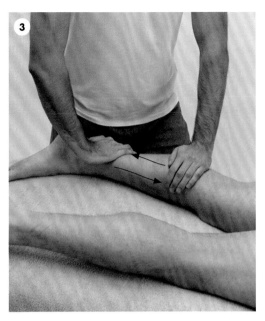

Alternate hand effleurage
3, 4 *Use both hands alternately to apply palm effleurage up and down the whole leg in a circular action.*

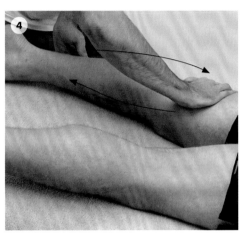

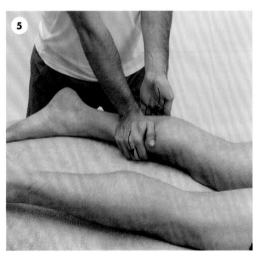

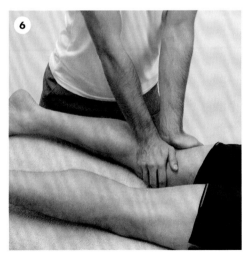

Palm pressure
5, 6 *Using both hands, apply alternating pressure up and down the whole leg.*

Continued overleaf

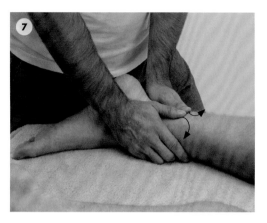

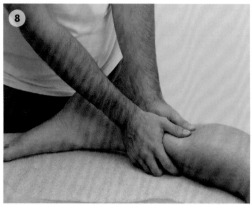

Thumb pressure on calf
7, 8 *Apply light circling pressure with the thumbs up the calf in three lines: inner, mid, and outer edge.*

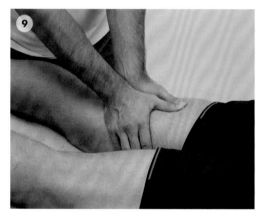

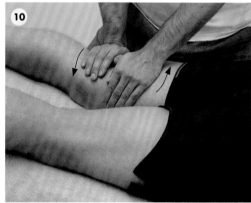

Thumb pressure on thigh
9 *Repeat the application of circling thumb pressure in three lines up the back of the thigh.*

Criss-cross rubbing
10 *Place both hands on the calf. Move them back and forth, moving up to treat the whole leg.*

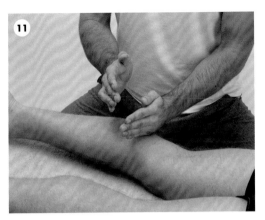

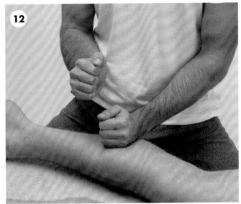

Hacking
11 *Use both hands alternately to hack up and down the whole leg.*

Pounding
12 *Use both closed fists alternately to pound up the whole leg. Continue, to include the gluteal muscles of the buttocks.*

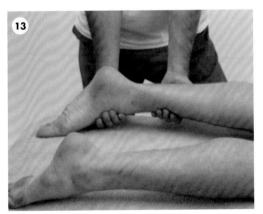

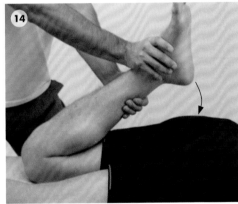

Quadriceps stretch
13, 14 *Place both hands under the ankle. Lift the lower leg to bend the knee, and move the heel back toward the buttocks. Apply gentle pressure for a count of three. Repeat three times.*

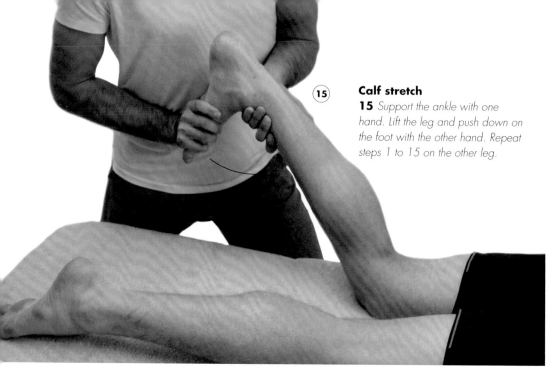

Calf stretch

15 *Support the ankle with one hand. Lift the leg and push down on the foot with the other hand. Repeat steps 1 to 15 on the other leg.*

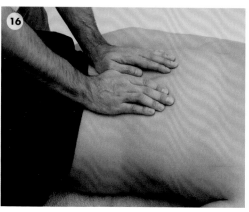

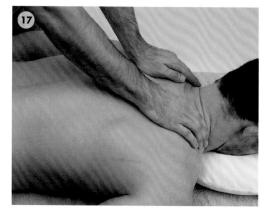

Back effleurage

16, 17 *Apply light effleurage strokes to the back in a heart shape. Use a brisk rhythm.*

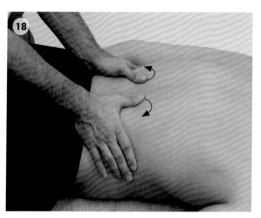

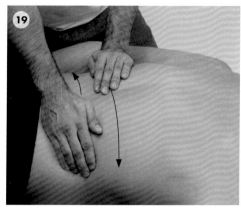

Thumb pressure
18 *Use both thumbs to apply light circling pressure on either side of the spine, working upward from the lower back.*

Criss-cross rubbing
19 *Rub across the back with criss-cross movements of the hands from the lower back to the upper back and down again.*

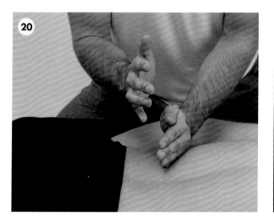

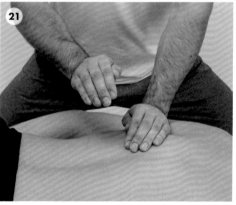

Hacking around the waist
20 *Use both hands to hack briskly across the waist area.*

Cupping
21 *Briskly apply cupping strokes across the whole back area, emphasizing the upper back to stimulate the lungs.*

Continued overleaf

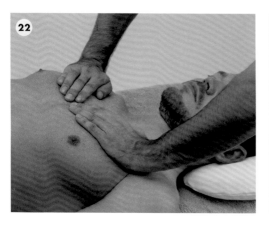

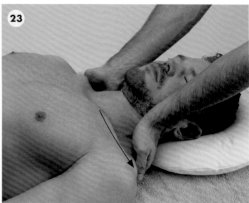

Chest effleurage

22, 23, 24 *With the receiver lying on his back, place both hands on the center of the upper chest. Apply gliding stokes, moving outward toward the shoulders. Cup the hands under the shoulder and bring the fingers back to the starting position.*

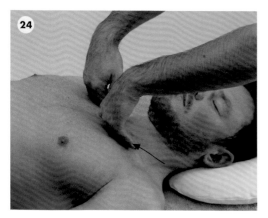

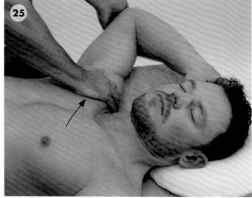

Pectoral muscle petrissage

25 *Bend one arm and place the receiver's hand under the head. Support the elbow with one hand. Apply pressure to the upper chest with the heel of the other hand, moving outward toward the shoulder. Repeat three times.*

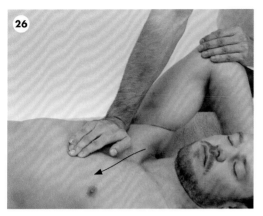

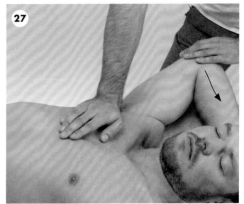

Pectoral stretch
26, 27 *Pressing down on the bent elbow, place the heel of the other hand on the side of the upper chest and exert diagonal pressure toward the center of the chest. Pressing down on the chest, move the elbow back toward the table. Repeat steps 25 to 27 on the other side.*

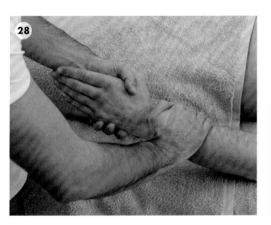

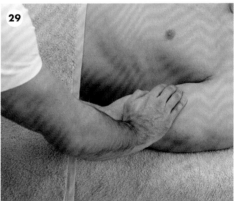

Arm effleurage
28, 29 *Keeping one hand in contact with the receiver's hand, use your other hand to apply effleurage strokes from wrist to shoulder.*

Continued overleaf

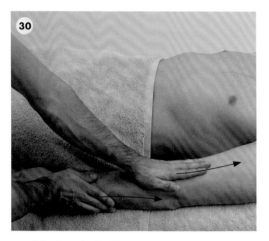

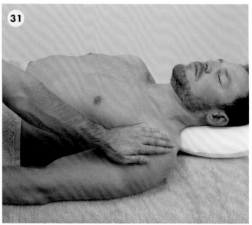

Double-handed effleurage

30, 31 *Continue effleurage from wrist to shoulder, using alternating strokes of both hands. Keep the rhythm brisk.*

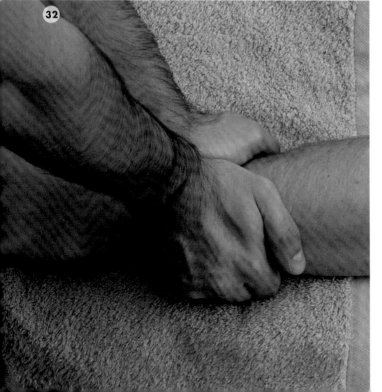

Compression

32, 33 *Enclose the wrist with both hands. Apply pressure using alternate hands, working from wrist to shoulder.*

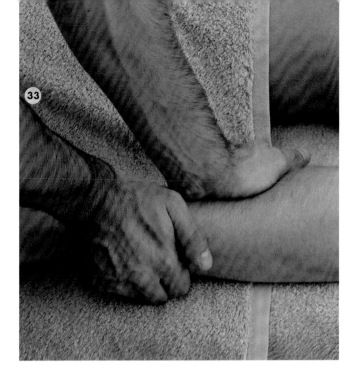

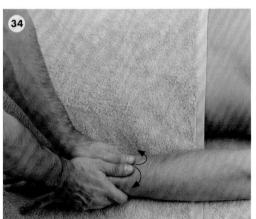

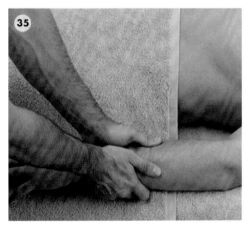

Thumb pressure

34, 35 *Make circling movements with the thumbs, using moderate pressure, working on the upper surface of the arm, from wrist to shoulder. Repeat steps 28 to 35 on the other arm.*

Continued overleaf

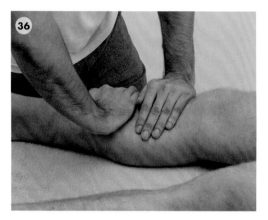

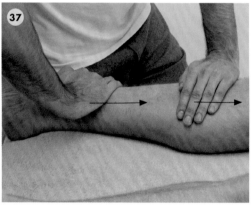

Lower leg double-handed effleurage
36 *Use both hands together to apply brisk effleurage strokes to the whole of the front of the leg, from ankle to thigh.*

Lower leg alternating hands effleurage
37 *Apply circulating effleurage strokes over the whole leg with alternating hands, in a brisk rhythm.*

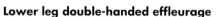

Criss-crossing
38 *Apply criss-crossing strokes across the front of the thigh.*

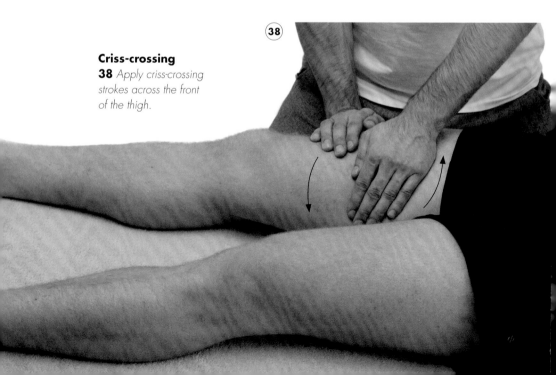

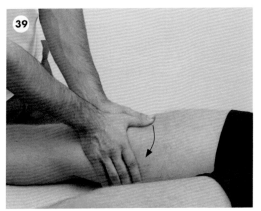

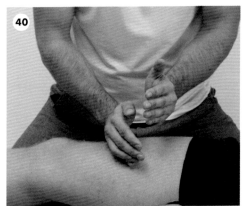

Thumb pressure
39 *Apply circulating thumb pressure up the thigh in three strips, from the knee to the top of the thigh.*

Hacking
40 *Apply hacking strokes to the thigh in a brisk rhythm.*

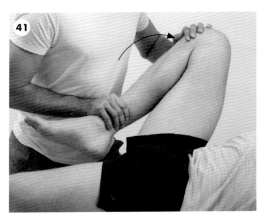

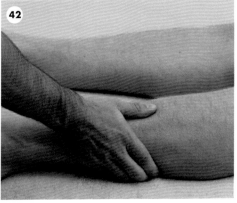

Hip mobilization
41 *Lift the leg with bent knee and move it back over the body. Apply pressure in the central position and then move the leg about 20 degrees to the side, and apply pressure. Move the leg to the other side and repeat.*

Thumb pressure
42 *Apply sliding thumb pressure up the outside of the lower leg on the muscle just below the bone. Repeat steps 36 to 42 on the other side.*

POST-EVENT MASSAGE
The emphasis of a post-event massage is on relaxing strokes and those that permit you to stretch muscles that have become overtight. These strokes also enhance lymphatic circulation, helping to prevent the development of muscle pain and stiffness. The rhythm should be slow. Essential oils that have a soothing or anti-inflammatory effect, such as geranium or lavender, can be added to your lubricant if this is acceptable to the person you are treating.

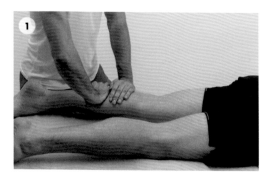

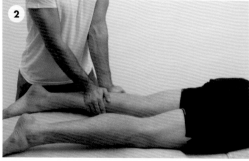

Whole-leg effleurage
1 *Apply double-handed effleurage strokes to the whole leg, from the ankle to the thigh.*

Compression
2 *Apply palm pressure using alternate hands to the calf muscle and back of the thigh.*

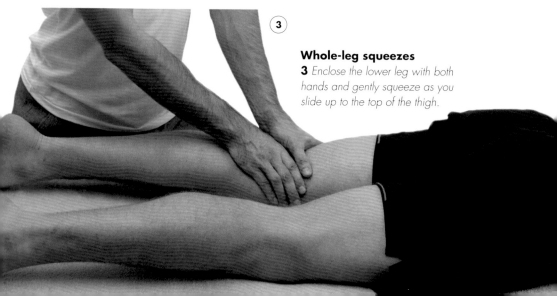

Whole-leg squeezes
3 *Enclose the lower leg with both hands and gently squeeze as you slide up to the top of the thigh.*

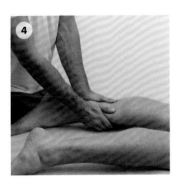

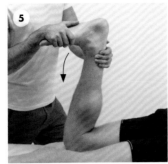

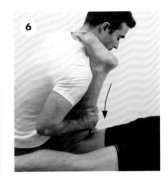

Thumb pressure

4 *Apply circulating thumb pressure in three strips up the lower leg and then do the same on the back of the thigh.*

Calf stretch

5 *Lift the lower leg so that the ankle is above the knee and then gently push down on the ball of the foot to stretch the calf muscle.*

Lower leg effleurage

6 *In the same position, support the foot against your shoulder and use both hands to apply effleurage strokes down the calf muscle. Repeat steps 1 to 6 on the other leg.*

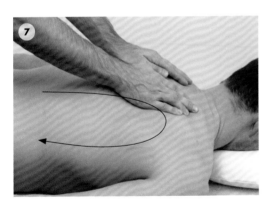

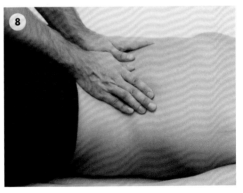

Back effleurage

7 *Apply effleurage strokes with both hands in a heart shape over the back.*

Pressure strokes

8 *Apply pressure on either side of the spine from the lower back to the upper back, first using your thumbs with a circulating action, then with the heels of your hands.*

Continued overleaf

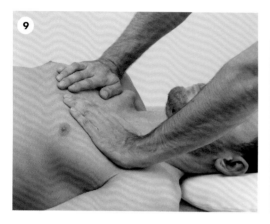

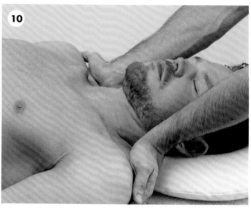

Chest effleurage
9 *With the receiver lying on his back, apply effleurage strokes to the chest at a slow rhythm. Bring the circulating stroke up the back of the neck. Use a light pressure.*

Shoulder press
10 *Apply fingertip pressure to the upper chest, working from the center toward the shoulder. Continue the previous movement by gently pressing onto the shoulder towards the feet.*

Back of the neck
11 *Place both hands at the back of the neck, one on either side of the spine. Use the tips of the fingers to draw the muscle up from the shoulders toward the base of the skull in an alternating rhythm.*

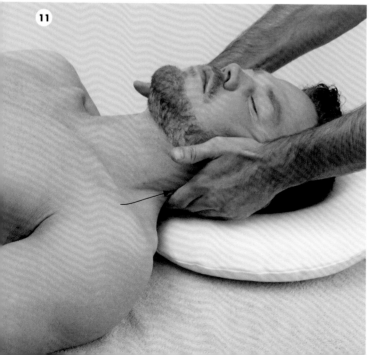

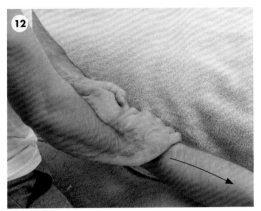

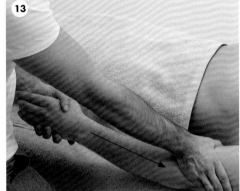

Arm effleurage
12 *Hold the receiver's hand and use your other hand to apply effleurage strokes up the length of the arm.*

Arm squeezes
13 *Apply a sliding and squeezing stroke up the arm.*

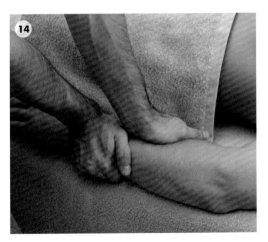

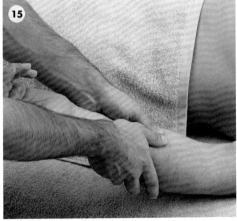

Arm compression
14 *Apply alternating compression strokes with the heel of the hand up the arm.*

Thumb pressure
15 *Apply circulating thumb pressure in three strips from wrist to shoulder. Repeat steps 12 to 15 on the other arm.*

Continued overleaf

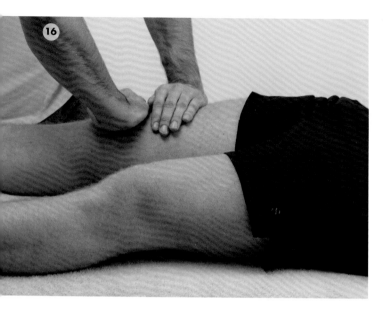

Whole-leg effleurage

Apply effleurage strokes up the whole leg in a slow rhythm.

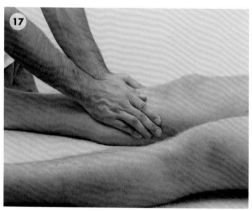

Leg squeezes

17 *Enclose the lower leg in both hands. Apply a gentle squeezing stroke up the whole leg.*

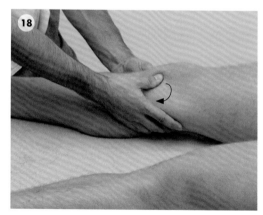

Thumb pressure

18 *Apply circulating thumb pressure from knee to thigh. Work up the thigh in three strips: center, outer, and inner thigh.*

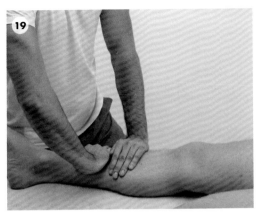

Thumb pressure around the knee
19 *Apply circulating thumb pressure around the knee area.*

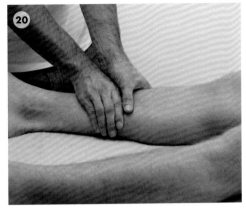

Lower-leg effleurage
20 *Apply double-handed effleurage strokes to the lower leg.*

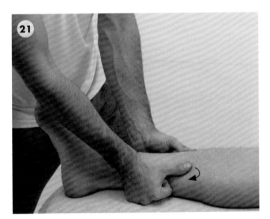

Thumb pressure on the lower leg
21 *Working on both sides of the lower leg simultaneously, apply circulating thumb pressure on either side of the shin bone.*

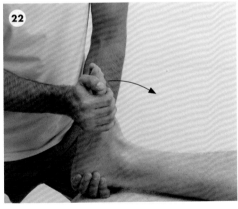

Calf stretch
22 *Support the heel in one hand and use your other hand to push the foot back. Do not attempt to achieve a full stretch but aim for a gentle pumping action. Repeat steps 16 to 22 on the other leg.*

SELF-MASSAGE TECHNIQUES

The reassurance and comfort provided by the hands of an experienced practitioner of massage provides unmatched therapeutic benefits. However, there are occasions when you need the help of a massage stroke to relieve pain or stiffness when there is no massage practitioner available. For example, you are at work and a headache develops or you notice painful stiffness in your shoulder. At times like this, it is useful to know that you can apply massage yourself to alleviate the problem.

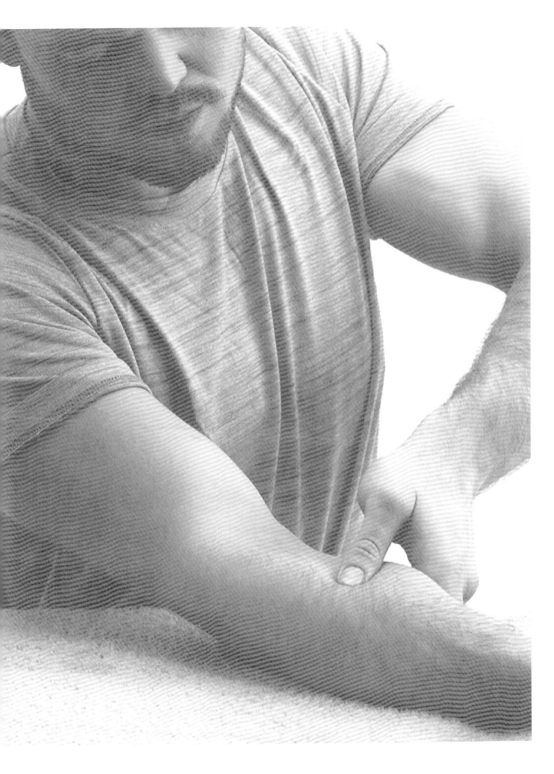

TEMPLES & JAW
The temples and the jaw are a common focus for tension. Steps 1 to 3 on this page are often effective in providing relief from headaches and can beneficially be performed with steps 4 to 6 in a longer sequence to alleviate tension in the jaw. These massages are best performed when sitting upright in a chair.

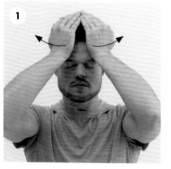

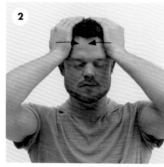

Pressure
1, 2 *Place the heels of both hands in the center of the forehead and drag them outward toward the temples. Use the heel of your hands to apply pressure to the temples.*

Fingertip massage
3 *Use the tips of your fingers to massage both temples in a circular motion, then do the same with your thumbs.*

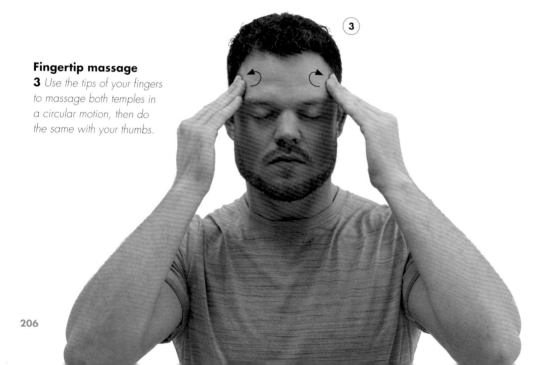

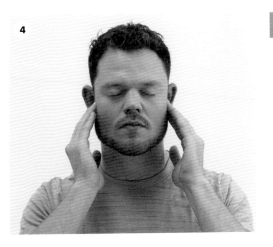

Although massage given by another person has many advantages over self-massage, when you massage yourself you are in full control of the pressure and duration of the stroke. You will instantly know when the contact is having the desired effect and can continue or cease as required.

Under the cheekbone
4 *Place your fingers on the upper part of the jaw under the cheekbone.*

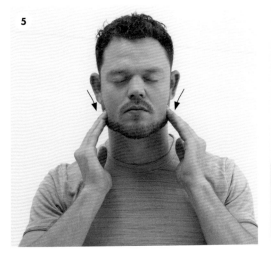

Sliding down
5 *Using medium pressure, slide your fingertips down to the angle of the jaw.*

Circling pressure
6 *Make circular movements with your thumbs to apply pressure under the cheekbones.*

BACK OF NECK & SHOULDERS

The muscles of the neck and shoulders can easily become stiff and painful as a result of unaccustomed exercise, including lifting and carrying or sporting activities. Massage can provide relief of tension in both areas. Sit in an upright chair to perform these massages.

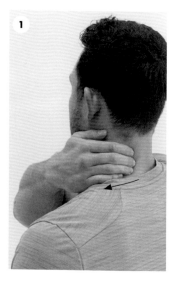

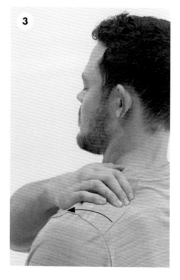

Neck pulls

1 *Cross your arm across your body and place your fingers on the near side of the spine. Use your fingers to pull the flesh toward the front of the neck. Repeat on the other side.*

Thumb circling

2 *Place your thumbs at the base of the skull and make circling movements.*

Shoulder pulls

3 *Cross your arm across your body. Hook your hand over your shoulder and pull the muscle forward. Repeat on the other side.*

Mental Relaxation

Self-massage can not only address specific aches and pains in the areas you can reach but also provide the opportunity for mental relaxation in your busy and perhaps stressful day. Taking the time to work on tense muscles also allows you to focus on the sensations that you are feeling here and now, rather than on your worries and fears. Whatever part of the body you are treating, you will also experience psychological benefits.

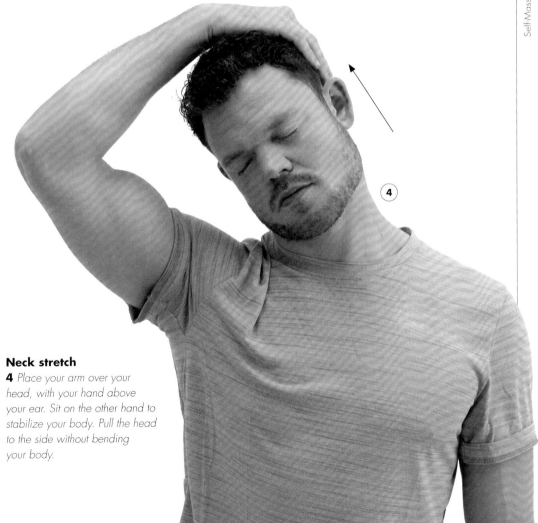

(4)

Neck stretch
4 *Place your arm over your head, with your hand above your ear. Sit on the other hand to stabilize your body. Pull the head to the side without bending your body.*

HANDS & FOREARMS
Muscle tension affecting the hands and arms is an increasingly common problem for those engaged in office or factory work, in which repetitive movements bring the risk of strain that in extreme cases can be disabling. Use this technique to relieve muscle tiredness and stiffness whenever you feel the need.

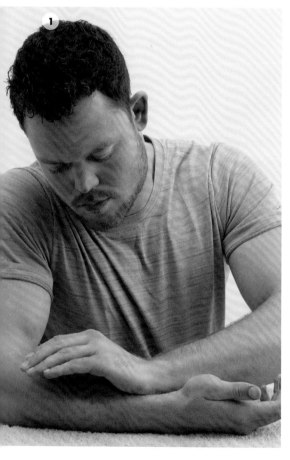

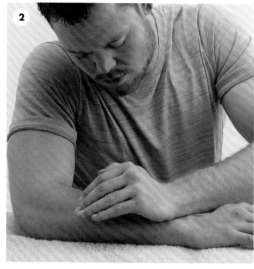

Inner-arm compression
1 *Resting your arm on a support with palm up, apply pressure with the heel of the other hand from wrist to elbow.*

Outer-arm compression
2 *Turn the arm palm downward and repeat, applying pressure on the top of the arm. Repeat steps 1 to 2 on the other arm.*

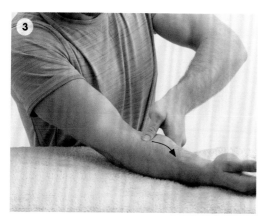

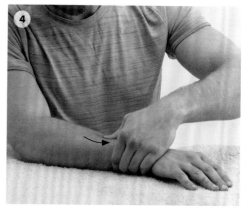

Thumb pressure—inner arm
3 *With the palm upward, apply circling pressure with your thumbs, working downward from just below the elbow toward the wrist.*

Thumb pressure—outer arm
4 *With the palm downward, apply circling pressure with the thumbs to the top of the arm from elbow to wrist. Repeat steps 3 and 4 on the other arm.*

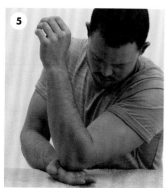

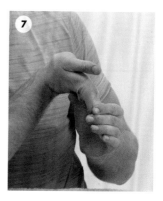

Pressure on the palm
5 *Use the point of your elbow to apply pressure in the center of the palm of the other hand. Repeat on the other hand.*

Finger pulls
6 *Pull each of the fingers of both hands, firmly but not too strongly.*

Wrist stretch
7 *Use your hand to push the fingers of the other hand back to extend the knuckles and the wrist. Hold for a count of three. Repeat on the other hand.*

CALF & FOOT

Use the techniques described here to relieve tiredness and strain, which can result from unaccustomed exercise of various kinds. For those who spend long periods standing, the feet, in particular, benefit from regular self-massage. To perform the massages on these pages, sit in an upright chair or stool.

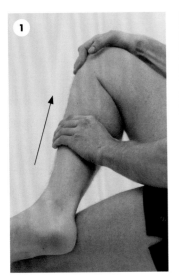 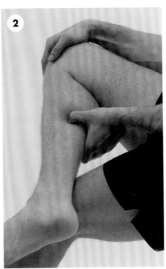 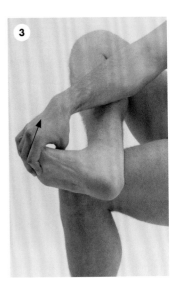

Calf pressure
1 *Cross one leg over the other with the ankle resting on the thigh. Enclose the calf with your hand and, applying pressure with the web between your thumb and fingers, slide up from the ankle to just below the knee.*

Calf squeezes
2 *Squeeze the muscle between your thumb and fingers, working up toward the knee.*

Calf stretches
3 *Gently ease the ball of the foot upward to stretch the calf muscle. Repeat steps 1 to 3 on the other leg.*

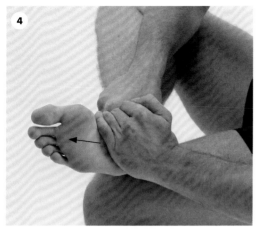

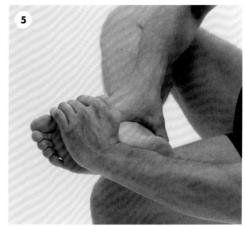

Heel-of-hand pressure

4, 5 *Sit with one foot on the other thigh. Supporting the ankle with one hand, apply pressure along the sole of the foot from the heel to the ball of the foot, using the heel of your hand.*

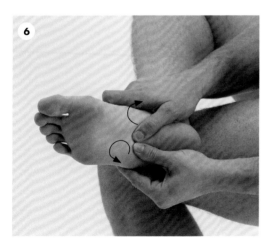

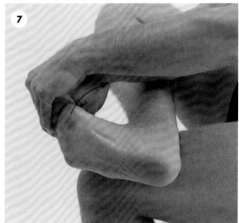

Thumb pressure

6 *Use both thumbs to apply circling pressure all over the sole of the foot.*

Foot stretch

7 *Grasp the toes and pull them upward to stretch the underside of the foot. Repeat steps 4 to 7 on the other foot.*

Taking It Further

You have learned the essential skills of massage and perhaps you are considering taking your interest to a new level. There are several directions in which you could go.

Massage training

For most people, the next step would be to enroll in a recognized massage course. You will find details of training organizations in the Resources section. In such courses you will learn how to refine your skills and how to conduct yourself in a professional context. You will also learn more about the therapeutic aspects of massage practice and be given a thorough background in human anatomy and physiology. You will need to check that the certificates offered meet the requirements of any job or career progression you are considering.

Other complementary therapies

Your interest in massage may lead you to develop your understanding of related complementary therapies. These could include aromatherapy—to extend your knowledge of the actions and uses of essential oils—and reflexology, to learn more about the benefits of foot massage. Learning about traditions from other cultures may also extend your practice. Shiatsu, Indian head massage, and Lomi Lomi Hawaiian massage are examples that you may wish to investigate.

Sports massage

Many massage practitioners decide to specialize in preventing and treating sports injuries. This requires extensive additional training provided by a dedicated course. You will learn how to treat damage and to boost rehabilitation following an injury, as well as receiving training in additional massage techniques.

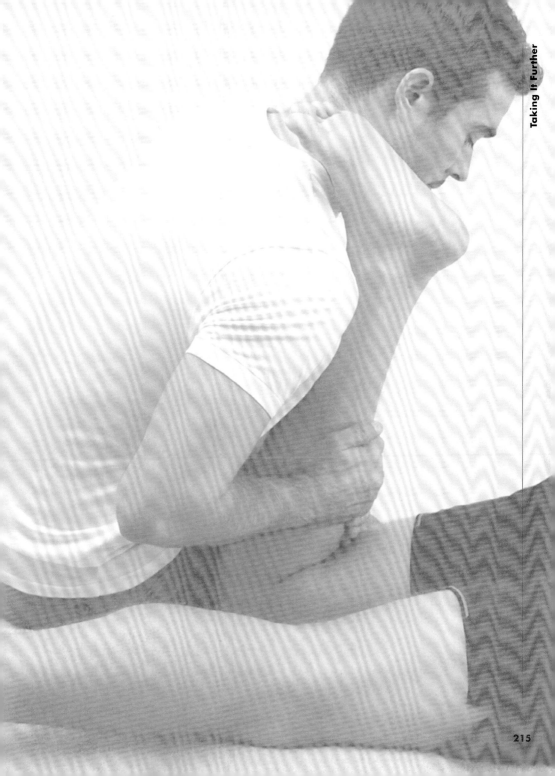

GLOSSARY

Acupressure

The ancient Chinese practice of using pressure of the thumb, finger, or other part of the body to stimulate the flow of vital energy throughout the body

Anma

The traditional form of Chinese massage from which the practice of Shiatsu is derived.

Aromatherapy

The use of essential oils derived from plants to provide physical and psychological benefits.

Ayurvedic medicine

The 3,000-year-old Indian system of healing, based on ideas described in the ancient Sanskrit text, the Ayurveda. It employs herbal medicines and special diets to treat illness and promote better health.

Carrier oil

A neutral oil, such as sunflower oil, used as a base to which essential oils may be added.

Compression

A form of massage stroke in which pressure is applied to muscles. Compression helps muscles to soften and lengthen and stimulates blood flow to the area.

Effleurage

A flowing massage stroke that is often used to initiate and end a massage session. Effleurage encourages relaxation.

Essential oil

Highly concentrated fragrant oil that can be derived from many different plants and flowers, used in aromatherapy. Such oils can be added to a carrier oil for use as a massage lubricant.

Friction

Massage strokes that involve firmly rubbing areas of the body to release muscle stiffness.

Grounding

The initial static contact to accustom the receiver of massage to the massage therapist's touch.

Indian head massage

A form of massage that employs a variety of rubbing strokes, often with scented oils.

Lactic acid

A by-product of muscle activity, produced when oxygen levels are depleted, and which can cause pain and stiffness in muscles. Massage therapists believe that massage can help to remove excess lactic acid from muscles.

Lubricant

A substance, usually an oil or cream, that is used in massage to allow the practitioner's hands to slide smoothly over the skin of the receiver of massage.

Lymphatic drainage

A specialized form of massage that aims to promote the flow of lymph through the lymphatic system.

Meridians

The channels in the body through which, according to traditional Chinese medicine, vital energy—chi—flows. Shiatsu and acupressure act on these channels to promote well-being.

Edema

The pooling of fluid in body tissues, usually resulting from poor circulation.

Palpation

The assessment of body tissues, primarily muscles, through touch to gauge their condition and determine appropriate treatment.

Percussion

Invigorating strokes that involve brisk tapping with different parts of the hand.

Petrissage

A group of medium-pressure strokes used to stretch muscle fibers and boost circulation.

Reflexology

A complementary therapy based on the idea that points on the foot relate to particular body systems. In reflexology, massage and manipulation of specific areas of the foot is said to benefit the functioning of the related body system or organ.

Shiatsu

A massage system, derived from the ancient Chinese practice of anma, which uses pressure on specific points in the body, known as tsubos, to enhance the flow of vital energy.

Swedish massage

A term commonly used to describe the massage system popularly thought to have been developed by the Swedish practitioner Per Henrik Ling. Nowadays, this form of massage is more commonly known as classic massage.

Tapotement

An alternative term for percussion strokes.

Vibration

A technique in which areas of muscle are moved gently but rapidly to produce a stimulating or relaxing effect.

USEFUL ADDRESSES

USA

American Massage Therapy Association
500 Davis St, Suite 900
Evanston
IL 60201
USA
amtamassage.org

Massage Therapy Foundation
500 Davis St, Suite 950
Evanston
IL 60201
USA
massagetherapyfoundation.org

US Sports Massage Federation
2156 Newport Blvd
Costa Mesa
CA 9262
USA

CANADA

Canadian Sport Massage Therapists Association (CSMTA)
1030 Burnside Road West
Victoria
British Columbia
V8Z 1N3
Canada
csmta.ca

UK

Complementary and Natural Healthcare Council (CNHC)
46–48 East Smithfield
London
E1W 1AW
UK
cnhc.org.uk

The Council for Soft Tissue Therapies (GCMT)
27 Old Gloucester St
London
WC1N 3XX
UK
gcmt.org.uk

Massage Training Institute (MTI)
PO Box 368
23 Lindsay Avenue
Hitchin
SG5 9DT
UK
massagetraining.co.uk

International Examining Board (ITEC)
itecworld.co.uk

Vocational Training Charitable Trust (VTCT)
vtct.org.uk

Complementary Therapists Association (CThA)
Second Floor, Chiswick Gate
598–608 Chiswick High Road
London
W4 5RT
UK
ctha.com

Federation of Holistic Therapies (FHT)
18 Shakespeare Business Centre
Hathaway Close
Eastleigh
SO50 4SR
UK
fht.org.uk

London School of Massage
455 Caledonian Rd
London
N7 9BA
UK

10 Bonnersfield Lane
Harrow
Middlesex
HA1 2JR
UK
londonschoolofmassage.co.uk

AUSTRALIA
Massage Association of Australia Ltd
2/1–5 Station St
Moorabbin
VIC 3189
Australia
maa.org.au

Massage and Myotherapy Australia
massagemyotherapy.com.au

Australian College of Sports Therapy (ACST)
Level 5, 131 Queen St
Melbourne
VIC 3000
Australia
sportstherapy.edu.au

INDEX

ACKNOWLEDGMENTS

The publisher would like to thank the following for permission to reproduce copyright material:

Alamy/Historical image collection by Bildagentur-online: 17.

Bridgeman Images/Kuhn-Regnier, Joseph (1873-1940)/Private Collection/The Stapleton Collection: 11.

Getty/DEA/G. DAGLI ORTI/Contributor: 14B; Werner Forman/Contributor: 13; Dorling Kindersley: 12; Genevieve Naylor/Contributor: 19; Julian Winslow: 67.

iStock/andresr: 55; KatarzynaBialasiewicz: 71BL; dcdebs: 69BG; deliormanli: 70T; dolgachov: 70B; imagestock: 85; jacoblund: 39; Lilkin: 68; najin: 95; nico_blue: 30B; OSTILL: 32T; pixdeluxe: 24T; robertprzybysz: 75; Squaredpixels: 38B; velllena: 83.

Shutterstock/Africa Studio: 66, 91L, 113; all_about_people: 6; Antonina Vlasova: 90R; BezierMagic: 56T, 88; Goran Bogicevic: 73; brovkin: 42T; Rommel Canlas: 18B; Chin Kit Sen: 60T; focal point: 27; goir: 69T; Hanzi-mor: 64; Image Point Fr: 24B; itor: 87BR; kazmulka: 91R; Elvira Koneva: 79; LAUDiseno: 4–5; lightwavemedia: 77, 81; Microgen: 185; NORUEN: 44, 52, 72; Hein Nouwens: 86L, 87T; nuwatphoto: 71BR; ostill: 2, 8, 21, 32B, 42B, 51, 54B, 56B, 58, 71TR; picturepartners: 87BL; PPVector: 34T; puhhha: 89; Robert Przybysz: 63; Giorgio Rossi: 18T; Benjavisa Ruangvaree: 92; Norjipin Saidi: 57T; Rostislav_Sedlacek: 23; sukiyaki: 9, 109L; Swapan Photography: 90L; Evgeniya Usynina: 28T; venimo: 36, 46, 48, 54T; Ivan Veselinovic: 30T; Vshivkova: 38T; wasanajai: 91C; wavebreakmedia: 22T, 25, 26–27, 53, 93; Mahathir Mohd Yasin: 86R.

All reasonable efforts have been made to trace copyright holders and to obtain their permission for the use of copyright material. The publisher apologizes for any errors or omissions in the list above and will gratefully incorporate any corrections in future reprints if notified.